ASSESSMENT OF PRIOR LEARNING
A PRACTITIONER'S GUIDE

MALCOLM DAY

SECOND EDITION

WITHDRAWN

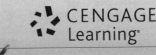

CENGAGE Learning

Brazil • Japan • Korea • Mexico • Singapore • Spain • United Kingdom • United States

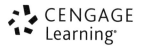
CENGAGE
Learning®

**Assessment of Prior Learning:
A Practitioner's Guide, 2e**

Malcolm Day

Publishing Director: Linden Harris

Commissioning Editor:
 Annabel Ainscow

Development Editor: Abigail Jones

Production Editor: Alison Cooke

Production Controller: Eyvett Davis

Marketing Manager: Lauren Mottram

Typesetter: Cenveo Publisher Services

Cover design: Adam Renvoize

For product information and technology assistance,
contact **emea.info@cengage.com**.

For permission to use material from this text or product,
and for permission queries,
email **emea.permissions@cengage.com**.

British Library Cataloguing-in-Publication Data
A catalogue record for this book is available from the British Library.

ISBN: 978-1-4080-6805-2

Cengage Learning EMEA
Cheriton House, North Way, Andover, Hampshire, SP10 5BE
United Kingdom

Cengage Learning products are represented in Canada by Nelson Education Ltd.

For your lifelong learning solutions, visit
www.cengage.co.uk

Purchase your next print book, e-book or e-chapter at
www.cengagebrain.com

Printed in Singapore by Seng Lee Press
1 2 3 4 5 6 7 8 9 10 – 15 14 13

BRIEF CONTENTS

CONTENTS

ACKNOWLEDGEMENTS

The Author would like to acknowledge the Canadian Association for Prior Learning Assessment(CAPLA). Also, the Clute Institute, USA who have agreed to the work of Day (2011 and 2012) being replicated in this text. The Author would also like to thank Debbie Hatfield, Professor Mark Gallupe, Carolyn Mann, and Dr Kaylash Algoo – their considerable knowledge of APL in the UK, Canada, the USA and Mauritius has made a unique contribution to this text.

Malcolm Day

Malcolm Day is registered with the UK Nursing and Midwifery Council as an Adult Nurse and a Practice Educator. He is a Fellow of the Institute for Learning and a Fellow of the Higher Education Academy. Malcolm has previously held university lectureships in nursing, community care, and care management. He was Lead Investigator to the:

- National Canadian APL Benchmarking Study, funded by Human Resources Development Canada;
- Canadian 'Technofile' APL project, which was funded by the Canadian Technology Human Resources Board in Ottawa;
- Canadian Adult Learner Friendly Institutions Study which, was funded by Human Resources Skills Development Canada.

Malcolm is the recipient of the following scholarships and awards:

- British Council Professional Exchange Award to examine Competence Based and Prior Learning Assessment within the Province of British Columbia, Canada.
- United Negro College Fund Special Programs Corporation (UNCFSP). Tertiary Linkages Project 11. Contract no. 674-C-00-03-00014-00 to develop and progress Recognition of Prior Learning (RPL) in 4 newly emerging universities of technology throughout South Africa.

Malcolm is currently a Lecturer in Adult Nursing and APL coordinator for the School of Nursing, Midwifery and Physiotherapy at Nottingham University and a Post Graduate Research Student at Sunderland University.

Dr Kaylash Allgoo

Dr Kaylash Allgoo is the Director of the Mauritius Qualifications Authority (MQA), the regulatory body for the Technical and Vocational Education and Training (TVET) sector in Mauritius. He is a Fellow to the Institute of Commercial Management and Honorary Fellow of the Organisation of Tourism and Hospitality Management, UK. Kaylash is also a member of the Management Committee of the Virtual University of the Small States of the Commonwealth (VUSSC) and Chairperson of the Transnational Qualifications Framework (TQF) Management Committee.

Serving as the Director of the MQA, he has successfully integrated the National Qualifications Framework in the Mauritian Education and Training System and developed the Mauritian Model for Recognition of Prior Learning in the TVET sector.

Kaylash is regularly invited to attend and contribute to several conferences and workshops both in Mauritius and internationally. His innovative approach to organizational excellence has gained him several prestigious awards including:

- Being elevated by the President of the Republic of Mauritius, as Officer of the Star and Key of the Indian Ocean (OSK) for Distinguished Services in the Education Sector; and
- The Knighthood award 'Chevalier dans L'Ordre des Palmes Academiques' by the French Government;
- Guest Professorship by Nanjing University.

Mark Gallupe

Mark is a Professor at Loyalist College, Belleville, Canada and has been an adult educator for 27 years. He is a professor and programme coordinator in the Social Service Worker Program and the Facilitator of Adult Learning/Teacher of Adults Program at Loyalist College in Belleville, Ontario, Canada.

Over the years he has worked closely and extensively with his friends and colleagues Paul Zakos and Rose Marie Reid on many projects involving adult learning practice, prior learning assessment, portfolio development and adult learner friendly institutions. Their work has taken them across Canada, South Africa and Chile.

Mark has participated as project facilitator in a national study on adult learning practices in Canada (2005–2007) entitled the Adult Learner Friendly Institutions (ALFICan) research project.

He was a co-founder and president of the Portfolio Development Centre. He co-authored several PLAR/RPL training manuals and is a lead facilitator in the PLAR Practitioner Training Program. Mark is a PLAR/RPL Advisor and Assessor at Loyalist College and a PLAR/RPL Assessor with Athabasca University in Alberta, Canada. For over 20 years he has attended and presented at the First Nations Technical Institute PLA Conference in Belleville.

Debbie Hatfield

Debbie is a senior lecturer in nursing at the University of Brighton and a registered nurse with the UK Nursing & Midwifery Council. She has extensive experience in pre-registration and post registration nurse education and has also worked as a trainer for NVQs in Care in the National Health Service. For seven years, until February 2012, she was the co-ordinator for Accreditation of Prior (Experiential) Learning at the School of Nursing and Midwifery at the University of Brighton. Debbie was also Deputy Chair of the AP(E)L Network, Southern England Consortium for Credit Accumulation and Transfer (SEEC) for three years until August 2012. She has presented and published in the field of flexible learning, in particular the role of work-related learning and skills.

Carolyn M. Mann

Carolyn M. Mann recently retired from Sinclair Community College. She brings a unique perspective as both practitioner and theorist to the field of prior learning. She began her career as an instructor assisting adults with the identification, articulation and documentation of college-level learning and advanced to creating and administering a comprehensive programme. During Carolyn's tenure Sinclair Community College was recognized for its leadership in assessing prior experiential learning. In 1998, Sinclair was selected as one of six institutions in the nation for a benchmarking study on Adult Learner Friendly Institutions. Carolyn has worked with numerous institutions to develop programmes in the United States and Canada. In addition, she has worked with the American Council on Education's (ACE) College Credit Recommendation Services programme, overseeing the Ohio office and more recently serving as one of eight National Coordinators.

PREFACE

The authors' experience of work based and experiential learning in North America and the United Kingdom (UK) has led to an increased awareness of the relationship between accreditation frameworks and the assessment and recognition of prior learning. In the UK experience of delivering National Vocational Qualifications (NVQs) and professional nursing diplomas and degrees has highlighted the importance of *credit exchange* or credential based models of prior learning assessment. This approach emphasizes '*products*' i.e. the achievement of competencies and the accreditation of prior certificated learning. Whereas, in North America, a more *developmental* approach towards assessment of prior learning is undertaken. This approach emphasizes '*process*' and the assessment and accreditation of prior experiential learning, which is often derived from work and community based experiences.

The North American preference for a more developmental approach is, in part, due to the early influence of the Council for Adult and Experiential Learning (CAEL) www.cael.org the work of the Canadian Association for Prior Learning Assessment (CAPLA) www.capla.ca and the ongoing influence of the First Nations culture, particularly the work the First Nations Technical Institute (Day, 2011) www.fnti.net Also, both the USA and Canada is governed by a federal system of government. There are no nationally agreed accreditation frameworks for post-compulsory education. The responsibility for ensuring currency and transferability of credentials rests with federal government bodies, while the delivery of credentials is the responsibility of state and provincial governments. The potential for mismatch is great, particularly as economic and cultural influences within each Canadian Province, and American State, are so diverse.

A study undertaken by CAPLA (Day, 2000a and 2000b) found that professional and occupational associations within North America are now showing an increased interest in the credit exchange, or credential based, model of assessment of prior learning. This is in part due to the need for occupations and professions to demonstrate that they can practice within a globally competitive market to an internationally acceptable standard e.g. see: Riffel (2006). As a consequence of this emerging interest a more eclectic or *complementary* approach towards assessment has been developing, where the best principles of practice from developmental *and* credit exchange models are now being used to enhance the validity and reliability of assessment decisions (Day, 2002). Similar approaches are now emerging in UK Universities, for example, in Schools of Nursing (Day, 2012).

In this text, international models for the delivery of prior learning assessment will be examined. This will include a discussion on the factors currently influencing assessment practice. Throughout the text examples will drawn from post compulsory and adult continuing education within Canada, Mauritius, USA and the UK.

THE PURPOSE OF THIS BOOK

This text is intended to encourage adult education students and newly appointed teachers, trainers and work based assessors to purposefully apply proven assessment theory to the practice of prior learning assessment. It identifies and discusses the basic principles and processes necessary for effective and systematic assessment of prior learning. These are well developed in Canada, the USA and the United Kingdom and are currently being developed within Mauritius. It is hoped that the assumptions, values, beliefs and practices espoused in this text will be applied in flexible, innovative and thoughtful ways that are respectful of the diverse backgrounds, interests and needs of adult learners.

DEFINING THE TERMS

Assessment

The Quality Assurance Agency for Higher Education (QAA) indicates that: '... *assessment describes any processes that appraises an individual's knowledge, understanding, abilities or skills*' (QAA 2006:4).

The QAA (2006:4) further indicate that there are many different forms of assessment, serving a variety of purposes. These include:

'*promoting student learning by providing the student with feedback, normally to help improve his/her performance*

    evaluating student knowledge, understanding, abilities or skills

    providing a mark or grade that enables a student's performance to be established. The mark or grade may also be used to make progress decisions

    enabling the public (including employers), and higher education providers, to know that an individual has attained an appropriate level of achievement that reflects the academic standards set by the awarding institution ... This may include demonstrating fitness to practise or meeting other professional requirements.'

Race (2006) states that the purpose of assessment is to:

- Guide students' improvement.
- Help students to decide which options to choose.
- Help students to learn from their mistakes or difficulties.
- Allow students to check out how well they are developing as learners.
- Allow students to make realistic decisions about whether they are up to the demands of a course or module.
- Add variety to students' learning.
- Determine fitness for entry to a programme.
- Help structure teaching and constructively align learning outcomes to assessments.
- Give feedback on the teachers ability to teach
- Classify or grade students.
- Translate intended learning outcomes into reality.
- Provide statistics for the course, or for the institution.
- Lead towards a licence to practice.
- Lead to appropriate qualifications.

Some of the above activities are *diagnostic* as they:

'... *provide an indicator of the learner's aptitude and preparedness for a program of study and identify possible learning problems*' (QAA, 2006:4).

For example, helping students to decide which options to choose.

Other assessment activities within the above list may be *formative*. The QAA (2006:35) indicates that formative assessment has:

'*a developmental purpose and is designed to help learners learn more effectively by giving them feedback on their performance and on how it can be improved and/or maintained*'.

Betts (2011) identifies five key strategies for formative assessment, which include:

- clarifying and understanding learning intentions and criteria for success;
- engineering effective classroom discussions, questions and tasks that elicit evidence of learning;
- providing feedback that moves learners forward;
- activating students as instructional resources for each other; and
- activating students as owners of their own learning.

Diagnostic and formative assessment is *learner focused* and is directly concerned with learning as a *process*. However, some of the activities listed by Race (2006) are terminal or *summative*. The QAA (2006:36) states that summative assessment is:

'*... used to indicate the extent of a learner's success in meeting the assessment criteria used to gauge the intended learning outcomes of a module or programme*'.

Summative assessment activities are *organizationally focused* and are directly concerned with learning as a *product* i.e. the achievement of an academic standard and/or fitness to practice. For example, Prozesky (2001) states that the purpose of a final examination is: '*To protect society*' He qualifies this statement by stating:

'*... we should only send out students who are* safe – *who know their work well enough not to harm anybody. One of the reasons for our final examination of students is to make sure that they are safe. Society expects us to do a good job*'

'Assessment' or 'Evaluation'?

These two words may have different meanings for people in different countries. For example, in the UK people 'assess' students to find out if they have learnt, and they 'evaluate' programmes, to see if they are effective. However, in the USA the two words are often used the other way around – they 'evaluate' students and 'assess' programmes. It doesn't matter which word you use, as long as you are clear about what you mean and what activities you and the learner will undertake.

Assessment and Recognition of Prior Learning

Assessment of Prior Learning or APL is defined as a systematic process that involves the identification, documentation, assessment and recognition of learning (i.e. skills, knowledge and values). This learning may be acquired through formal and informal study including work and life experience, training, independent study, volunteer work, travel, and hobbies and family experiences. Recognition of prior learning can be used toward the requirements of education and training programmes; occupational and/or professional certification; labour market entry; and organizational and human resource capacity building (CAPLA, 2000).

One of the difficulties encountered in trying to understand assessment of prior learning is the range of acronyms that are often used by different people, and in different countries. For example, in the United States it is known as Prior Learning Assessment or PLA (Keeton, 2000). In Canada it is known as Prior Learning Assessment and Recognition or PLAR (Blower, 2000). In South Africa and Australia it is known as Recognition of Prior Learning or RPL (Flowers and Hawke, 2000; Harris, 2000).

In the UK, it is known as AP(E)L, this term is generally used as an all-encompassing term to include prior *certificated* learning, as well as prior *experiential* learning (SEEC, 1995). This term includes Accreditation of Prior Achievements (APA). The claimant exchanges proof of past achievements in the workplace for unit credits within a nationally agreed framework (Simosko, 1992). AP(E)L in the UK also includes the Accreditation of Prior Certificated Learning (APCL) that is, learning for which certification has been awarded by an educational institution or another education or training provider. AP(E)L also includes the Accreditation of Prior Experiential Learning (APEL); this refers to un-certificated learning gained from experience.

Within this text the term: '*Assessment of Prior Learning*' will be used as a definition to encompass all of the above terms, and the acronym '*APL*' will be used with this specific meaning in mind.

Also, in this text assessment of prior learning has been differentiated from the process of '*accreditation*' or '*recognition*' of prior learning as it is the practice of prior learning assessment which is the focus of this publication. The methods that might be used to assess prior learning include assessment of educational documents; portfolio review; demonstration or challenge processes (e.g. written/oral examinations, projects, assignments, performance observation, skill demonstrations, simulations and product assessments); standardized tests and programme review.

APL Practitioner

For the purpose of this text an APL Practitioner is defined as an individual who utilizes learner-focused activities to diagnose and formatively or summatively assess an individual's prior learning, either for academic credit or recognition of competence, using the goals and methods outlined above. This definition includes the work of the APL Adviser. It also includes the work of the APL Assessor, who is often but not exclusively, a subject matter expert from faculty. It may also include the work of the APL Coordinator, if he or she is directly involved in the guidance and assessment of individual candidates, or groups of candidates. In this text, the practice of prior learning assessment in Canada, Mauritius, the UK, and the USA will be examined.

THE CONTENTS OF THIS BOOK

Chapter 1. This introductory chapter is written by Malcolm Day and describes the concept of prior learning assessment and its theoretical underpinnings. It discusses the potential benefit of APL for learners, employers and education institutions. It also describes the relationship of APL to the establishment of a credit based system for the curriculum, and the factors which might influence the development of this. Finally, this chapter identifies emergent guidelines for practice and how these are being used to resolve issues currently influencing the APL process.

Chapter 2 also written by Malcolm Day examines the role of the APL practitioner, drawing upon the original work of the Canadian Association for Prior Learning Assessment (Day, 2000a, 2000b, 2001a and 2001b) and newly emerging benchmarks for practice in the UK to clarify the role of the APL advisor and assessor (Day, 2011).

Chapter 3 written by Debbie Hatfield focuses upon the definitions in chapters one and two to explore the history of APL in nursing, within the United Kingdom (UK). The ramifications of moving nurse education into higher education and the emergence of new curricula which explicitly invite APL for pre-registration nursing are discussed.

Chapter 4 written by Mark Gallupe examines the practice of APL within a human service programme at a community college in the province of Ontario, Canada. A description of the process that learners go through when seeking recognition or their prior learning is presented and an in-depth case study of the developmental or holistic approach towards APL is discussed.

Chapter 5 Written by Carolyn Mann describes the use of APL within the US Community College system, its history and methodological development.

Chapter 6 written by Kaylash Algoo offers a detailed analysis of the Mauritian model for APL. It highlights the factors that have triggered the implementation of APL within the Mauritian Education and

Training system and identifies the difficulties and tensions that have underpinned the establishment and development of APL within the Mauritian context.

Chapter 7 – the final chapter is written by Malcolm Day – discusses in detail how emergent benchmarks for the practice of APL relate to the ongoing career of the APL practitioner and how they might be used to support the practitioner's continuing professional development.

HOW TO USE THIS BOOK

The reader can, if he or she wishes, participate in a series of *Key Learning Activities* . These activities will enable him or her to reflect upon, and continuously improve, his or her own practice of prior learning assessment. A sample Learning Diary that will help you to record your answers to these key learning activities is given in Appendix One. Feedback on the key learning activities is given in Appendix Two. A glossary of terms is given at the back of the book.

Malcolm Day

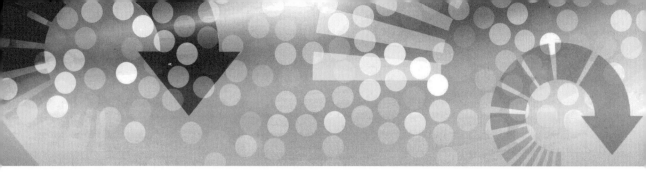

CHAPTER 1
WHAT IS ASSESSMENT OF PRIOR LEARNING?

This introductory chapter will describe the concept of Assessment of Prior learning (**APL**) and its theoretical underpinnings. It will discuss the potential benefit of APL for learners, employers and education institutions. It will also describe the relationship of APL to the establishment of a credit based system, and the factors which might influence the development of this. Finally, this chapter will identify emerging benchmarks for practice, and how these are being used to resolve issues which are currently influencing the APL process.

At the end of this Chapter, the reader will be able to:

● Describe what is meant by *Assessment of Prior Learning (APL)*.

● Outline the educational principles which underpin APL practice.

● Identify the benefits of APL for learners, employers and education institutions.

● Identify factors that are influencing the development of credit based systems.

● Identify possible guidelines, standards and benchmarks for APL practice.

WHAT IS ASSESSMENT OF PRIOR LEARNING?

Assessment of Prior Learning , or APL, is the general term used for the award of academic credit on the basis of learning that has occurred at some time in the past. This learning may have come about as the result of a programme of study, or as the result of experience gained at work or during voluntary activities, in the home or during leisure pursuits.

The credit that may be awarded by an education institution, on the basis of prior learning, may take the form of access or entry into a programme of study. It may take the form of exemption or advanced standing within a course of study. It might also involve certification or part credit towards an academic award.

The type and amount of credit that is awarded is based on certificates the learner has gained which demonstrate that learning has already been assessed, or it may take into account learning from experience. In this case credit is awarded for learning that can be demonstrated, not for the experience itself but for the learning that has arisen as a result of this experience.

This credit is considered to be of equal standing to that awarded to others who have followed a traditional course or programme of study.

Assessment of Prior Learning is of particular value to adult learners wishing to return to formal education, or to reduce the overall time spent on a programme or course of study. Adult learners wishing to seek credit via APL can do so on the basis of learning acquired at work, through voluntary work or from leisure activities. They may also do this on the basis of non-certificated learning from self-directed study, certificated learning from other educational institutions and certificated work-based learning.

Although APL can be used as a means of access or entry into educational institutions, the ways in which prior learning is now being used by learners is becoming increasingly varied. For example, prior learning may be assessed and used for access to a programme of education and training, for exemption from modules or units within programmes of education and training or the award of a qualification or credential.

Within Australia and the UK, APL has particularly been developed within the context of competence based education, for example, in the UK National Vocational Qualifications or **NVQs**, and more recently the new **QCF** Awards, Certificates and Diplomas. The assessment of existing competence, regardless of how or where this competence was achieved, is a fundamental principle of these vocationally related courses. The same principle is also fundamental to the practice of prior learning assessment.

Assessment of Prior Learning is a systematic process that involves the identification, documentation, assessment and recognition of learning. This learning may be acquired through formal and informal study including work and life experience, training, independent study, volunteer work, travel, and hobbies and family experiences. This learning can be used towards the requirements of education and training programmes, occupational and/or professional certification (CAPLA, 2000).

Challis (1993) states that the process of PLA includes: (1) the identification of learning, wherever it has taken place; (2) the selection of that learning that is relevant to an outcome, career or occupation; (3) demonstration of the **validity** and appropriateness of the learning; matching learning outcomes to those within a chosen accreditation framework; (4) assessment of evidence against criteria to ensure validity of the claimed learning; and (5) accreditation within a recognized accreditation framework.

Historically, two contrasting models for APL have emerged since the 1970s (Butterworth, 1992). Firstly, the *credit exchange model*. This has been used, for example, within competency based frameworks such as NVQs. Here, the learner identifies areas of a programme that they have achieved, and then offers evidence of these past achievements contained within a portfolio. Credit is awarded if the assessor and verifier agree that evidence contained within the portfolio proves possession of competence.

Secondly, the *developmental model*, which emphasizes the use of documentary evidence supported by reflective commentary. The learner's reflection is supported by discussions with a tutor. The purpose of these discussions is to support the learner's personal and professional development. The assessor judges both the evidence and the reflective commentary in the portfolio before recommending that academic credit should be awarded.

Several academics have argued that the credit exchange model is limiting, for example, Trowler (1996) has stated that it is derived from a behavioural model of learning and has no place in higher-level learning. Butterworth (1992) has taken this argument forward and explained that the developmental model provides a more legitimate pedagogy for higher education as it assists the learner to undertake an analysis of their own practice and to increase their professional expertise. This view is currently supported by Andersson (2006:34) who states the purpose of the developmental approach is to: '... *inform and change the continuing learning process*'. It is also supported by Popova–Gonci (2009) who in proposing building blocks for the US PLA community states that we should: '... *celebrate PLA as a learning process ...*'.

A study by Flemish researchers (Swegers *et al.*, 2009) has identified two types of APL portfolio the *recognition* portfolio and the *acknowledgement* portfolio. The recognition portfolio mainly fulfils a formative function, while the function of the acknowledgement portfolio is primarily summative. However Swegers *et al.*, indicate that the processes involved in developing either are *not* mutually exclusive. This suggests (perhaps) that a more integrated approach to APL is now emerging.

APL AND ADULT LEARNING

APL originally started in the USA, in the 1970s, as a research project entitled '*The Cooperative Assessment of Experiential Learning*'. From this project, in 1974, the Council for Adult and Experiential Learning (**CAEL**) was formed under the leadership of Dr Morris Keeton who indicates that:

> *CAEL was founded on two rather simple commonsense ideas: that what a learner knows and can do should be recognized appropriately no matter how or where it was learned and that hands-on experience of things being learned about and worked with can enhance that learning.*
>
> Keeton (2000:47)

Keeton's views are consistent with those expressed by early adult learning theorists, such as Carl Rogers (1969) and Malcolm Knowles (1980) – see Figure 1.1 (below).

FIGURE 1.1 The beliefs of two early adult learning theorists

Carl Rogers (1969)

- All human beings have a natural potential to learn;
- Significant learning occurs when the learner perceives the relevance of the subject matter;
- Learning involves a change in self-organisation and self-perception;
- Learning that threatens self-perception is more easily perceived and assimilated when external threats are at a minimum;
- Learning occurs when the self is not threatened;
- Much significant learning is acquired by doing;
- Learning is facilitated when the learner participates responsibly in the learning process;
- Independence, creativity and self-reliance are all facilitated when self-criticism, and self evaluation is integrated into the learning process;
- Much social useful learning is learning the process of learning and retaining an openness to experience, so that the process of change may be incorporated into the self.

Malcolm Knowles (1980)

- The adult learner is self directive;
- For the adult learner, experience becomes an exceedingly rich resource in learning;
- Adults learn from the problems with which they are confronted, and which they regard as relevant;
- Adult learners are more problem centred than subject centred.

Also, Kasworm and Marienau (1997:7) have established five principles for the assessment of adult learning. These include:

Recognizes multiple sources of knowing, that is, learning that occurs from interaction with a wide variety of informal and formal knowledge sources.

Recognizes and reinforces the cognitive, conative and affective domains of learning.

Focuses on adults' active involvement in learning and assessment processes, including active engagement in self-assessment.

Embraces adult learners' involvement in and impact on the broader world of work, on those contexts, family, and community.

Accommodates adult learners' increasing differentiation from one another given diversity among adult learners' varied life experiences and education.

Kasworm and Marienau (1997:7)

Each of the above approaches towards adult learning and the assessment of adult learning are consistent with the theory and practice of experiential learning, which emphasizes experience as a foundation for learning and knowledge production.

Typically, experiential learning theory is concerned with transforming experience thus: experience, plus reflection, equal learning and the acquisition of new knowledge. This is characterized in Kolb's experiential learning cycle, which describes the four stages of experiential learning – see Figure 1.2 (below).

However, many educationalists indicate that there is a dearth of systematic and empirical evidence to support an underpinning pedagogy for APL. For example Evans (2000:49) suggests that the evolution of APL has been based on: *'happenstance, coincidences and flukes of timing'*. Further, Joosten–Ten Brinke *et al.* (2008) have indicated that PLA literature is mainly descriptive and in order to learn more about the quality of PLA it is important to put PLA on the empirical research agenda. While Scott (2010) indicates that the number of empirical studies that test the assumption behind APL practice remain low.

Furthermore, there is a claim that much of the literature concerning APL appears to be overwhelmingly promotional, as it is often only the advocates of APL that write about the benefits of this type of assessment methodology, particularly with regard to the use of PLA as a form of social redress (Andersson and Harris, 2006).

However, much of the work associated with APL is based on accepted theory that is derived from a humanistic view of adult learning.

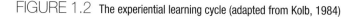

FIGURE 1.2 The experiential learning cycle (adapted from Kolb, 1984)

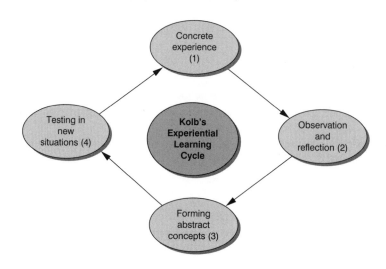

THE BENEFITS OF APL

According to the literature assessment of prior learning has three major benefits for the adult learner. *Firstly*, economic. For example, Scott (2010: 438) indicates that APL saves both time and money as individuals do not have to repeat learning that has already been undertaken. Also, Motaung (2009:78) states:

> *One way adult learners can accelerate their academic programmes, thereby saving time and money, is to seek out opportunities to gain recognition for learning acquired formally, informally, or non-formally.*
>
> Motaung (2009:78)

Secondly, APL is seen to be beneficial as a learning process. For example, Peruniak and Powel (2007) highlight the importance of APL in encouraging reflection on past learning as a mechanism to gain access to, advanced standing in, or course equivalency within the mainstream curriculum of post-secondary education. Also, Stevens *et al.* (2010) highlight the importance of the APL process as a mechanism for transformative learning. They state:

> *... there is no reason why the process of portfolio development needs to be limited to the awarding of college credit. It may be possible to adapt the process – the emphasis on reflection, writing, critical questioning, peer feedback – to other practice settings, settings in which the aim is to encourage transformative learning.*
>
> Stevens et al. (2010)

Thirdly, APL is often regarded as a way for underprivileged and marginalized members of society to improve their lives and career prospects. For example, Motaung (2009:78) states:

> *In South Africa the Recognition of Prior Learning (RPL) was conceptualized to address issues of social justice. The concept intended to increase the participation rate of historically disadvantaged groups in higher education ...*
>
> Motaung (2009:78)

Allgoo *et al.* (2012:19) summarize the benefits of APL to learners and employers as follows:

Benefits to Learners
... helps individual learners

   i) to ease the transition from informal and non-formal to formal learning by enabling the learners to value their achievements and to recognise the importance of their learning through experience;
   ii) to plan for further learning and personal/career development;
   iii) to gain entry to a programme of study (if they do not have the normal entry qualifications);
   iv) to obtain credit towards a programme of study thereby shortening the period of study;

Benefits to Employers
... can support training and staff development strategies of employers by:

   i) Increasing motivation and interest in workplace practice on the part of the employee/learner;
   ii) Reducing the amount of time needed to complete a qualification and therefore requiring less time away from the workplace;
   iii) Improving employee retention and preventing duplication of training.

THE PRINCIPLES UNDERPINNING APL PRACTICE

Assessment of prior learning is a process of continuous assessment that may involve *formative* (diagnostic) as well as *summative* (terminal) assessment (see preface). This may include assessment of educational documents; portfolio review; demonstration or challenge processes (e.g. written/oral examinations, projects, assignments, performance observation, skill demonstrations, **simulations** and product assessments);

standardized tests and programme review. In order to demonstrate rigor, the assessment process must be *valid, reliable and sufficient.*

- **Validity:** assessment should be based upon the required outcomes or competencies, and their associated criteria. Assessment is said to be valid if the assessor refers only to the stated criteria.
- **Reliability**: is concerned with the consistency of assessment. The degree to which an assessor's opinion may match that of another assessor in the same situation, with a similar adult learner using the same criteria.
- **Sufficiency**: in order that an assessment may be deemed to be sufficient adult learners must be able to demonstrate that all criteria within each of the specified outcomes have been met, including any necessary underpinning knowledge and understanding, where appropriate.

Evidence for APL must also be:

- **Current**: up-to-date.
- **Authentic**: the individual's own work.

In order that a College or University might successfully assess an individual's prior learning it must work within a credit based system that clearly defines the following:

- *credit*: a means of quantifying any learning that has been achieved;
- *level indicators*: of the demand, complexity and depth of study undertaken by the learner;
- *level descriptors*: statements describing the expectations of each level of study;
- *learning outcomes*: statements that describe what a learner should know, understand and/or be able to do;
- *assessment criteria*: statements that are used to demonstrate that learning outcomes have been achieved;
- *notional learning time*: the length of time that will be taken, on average, to achieve the learning outcomes;
- *module or units of learning*: a *self-contained* 'block' of learning which make up a course or programme of study.

For example, the above principles underpinning the Qualifications and Curriculum Framework or **QCF**. This is a newly emerging credit based system for recognizing skills and qualifications within England, Wales and Northern Ireland.

The QCF does this by awarding credit for qualifications that are made up of individual units. Each unit has a credit value. This value specifies the number of credits that can be gained by learners who complete that unit.

Within the QCF every unit and qualification has a credit value and a level. One credit represents ten notional hours of learning, showing how much time the average learner would take to complete the unit or qualification.

Within the QCF each qualification has a level of difficulty from Entry level at the bottom to Level 8 at the top. At Levels 1 to 3 there are three different sizes of qualification:

- Awards (1 to 12 credits)
- Certificates (13 to 36 credits)
- Diplomas (37 credits or more)

Levels 4 to 8 of the QCF represent the types of work undertaken in Higher Education i.e. the Framework for Higher Education qualifications or FHEQ. For example:

Level 3 is typical of the learning expected of entry qualification for HE
Level 4 is typical of the learning expected of the first part of HE
Level 5 is typical of the learning expected of a foundation degree
Level 6 is typical of the learning expected of the last part of a bachelors degree
Level 7 is typical of the learning expected of a masters degree
Level 8 is typical of the learning expected of a doctorate

Within the QCF credit is awarded to individuals who are able to show that they have successfully completed a unit, module or qualification. To do this, they need to meet all of the learning outcomes of that unit, module or qualification.

Also, within the QCF the credit value indicates the *amount* of learning achieved as well as the level of *difficulty*. Once the learner has successfully achieved all of the learning outcomes they can be awarded the full credit value for that block of learning. This credit value is based on *notional hours of learning* (usually 1 credit = ten hours).

ESTABLISHING CREDIT VALUE: An FHEQ module that has been designed to meet level descriptors at Level 4, which consists of 150 hours of learning, will be assigned a credit value of 15 credits at Level 4. Therefore once an individual has successfully demonstrated they have met the learning outcomes of this module they can be awarded 15 credits at Level 4 of the FHEQ – Source: QAA (2006)

Within the QCF an individual can progress by *accumulating* the credit value of modules or units they have completed successfully. Also, individuals can *transfer* the credits they have been awarded – either within the same college or university – or when moving from one institution to another. However, some institutions may describe credit as either general or specific to a particular programme. This will have important implications if an individual wants to transfer the credit they have been awarded in one programme, to a programme in a different subject area.

A similar credit framework for Scotland also exists – see http://www.scqf.org.uk/ However the Scottish Credit and Qualifications Framework (SCQF) has 12 levels ranging from Access at SCQF Level 1, up to Doctorate at Level 12. The credit that can be accrued by an individual within the SCQF is also determined by level outcomes and level descriptors as well as the number of notional hours of learning undertaken, which is also based on the formulae of 1 credit = ten hours.

Colleges and universities within England, Wales, Northern Ireland and Scotland can provide individuals with a record of their accumulated credits. This is usually in the form of a *transcript*, which can be a useful document for individuals who want to take a break from learning and return to study later, or transfer their credits. Therefore, in the UK an individual might gain a qualification partly through *credit accumulation*, partly through *credit transfer*, and partly through the submission of APL evidence; or a combination of each of these. Finally, it is important to remember that it is the achievement of learning outcomes that is critical to the award of credit, not how or where the learning took place, or the method that was used to assess the individual.

Credit based systems similar to the principles already discussed have also been developed within South Africa and Mauritius. The South African National Qualifications Framework (NQF) came into being through the South African Qualifications Authority (SAQA) in 1995 and consists of Eight Levels. Level 1 of the NQF makes up the general education and training band; Levels 2 to 4 make up the Further Education and Training Band; and Levels 5 to 8 make up the Higher Education and Training Band. Further information about SAQA can be obtained from http://www.saqa.org.za The National Credit framework for Mauritius is discussed in Chapter 6.

FACTORS INFLUENCING THE DEVELOPMENT OF CREDIT BASED SYSTEMS

Many countries are looking for better ways of educating their people and organizing their education and training systems so that they might gain the edge in an increasingly competitive economic global environment. For example, the current aim of UK Government policy is to increase participation in post-compulsory education and training, to raise the overall skill level of their workforce. This policy is driven by the need to make the workforce more competitive in the global economy (Lenney and Ponton, 2007).

Within South Africa the policy aim is also to widen participation in post compulsory education and to include groups who have previously been under-represented, including black and ethnic minorities. This is partly driven by the need to improve social cohesion as South Africa emerges from the effects of apartheid but also to: *'enhance the functional and intellectual capability of the nation, thereby increasing chances for success in the global community' (SAQA, 2012).* The rationale for a credit based system is eloquently summarized by SAQA (2012) who state:

> *When learners know that there are clear learning pathways which provide access to, and mobility and progression within education, training and career paths, they are more inclined to improve their skills and knowledge, as such improvements increase their employment opportunities.*
>
> *SAQA (2012)*

Within Canada and the USA there are no nationally agreed accreditation frameworks for post compulsory education. The responsibility for ensuring currency and transferability of credentials rests with federal government bodies, while the delivery of credentials is the responsibility of state and provincial governments. As a consequence many community colleges have now developed there own credit frameworks – often influenced by national associations such as the Council for Adult and Experiential Learning (CAEL). Examples of how prior learning is assessed within Canada is given in Chapter Four. The work of CAEL and its influence on APL policy and practice is outlined later in this chapter.

However, unlike other pedagogical approaches, the practice of APL has not been developed or refined, through a process of systematic and rigorous enquiry This has led to much scepticism, as well as resistance towards the practice of within Colleges and Universities. Perhaps its not surprising therefore, that APL has been subject to much controversy, for example, there is ongoing debate concerning the relative value of learning gained outside the formal education system. This debate serves to reinforce existing tensions between employers, students and education providers, and creates barriers for individuals wishing to have their non-formal learning recognized and accredited. This phenomena is often referred to as *'academic gate keeping'*. This phenomenon was first described by Trowler (1996) and is an indicator of the power relationship which exists between the learner and faculty member, which can influence the APL process.

The tensions underpinning APL practice are described by Day (2011:20) and are summarized in Figure 1.3 below:

FIGURE 1.3   The tensions underlying APL practice in higher education

Objectivity *versus* Bias i.e. academics have higher expectations of PLA students than those who are attending taught courses, and are therefore biased in the way they assess non-institutional learning.

Equality *versus* Elitism i.e. Professions are now considering alternative forms of entry for individuals with vocational qualifications. There is a concern that this may lead to a drop in standards.

Internalization *versus* Alienation of learning i.e. there is a belief that PLA activity may become so focussed on meeting assessment outcomes that learners become alienated from the learning they have experienced.

Quality *versus* Excessive surveillance i.e. the need to quality assure assessment outcomes must be balanced against the purpose of the assessment, as well as the desire for utility.

Congruence *versus* Discord i.e. if academics cannot agree that PLA is a systematic and rigorous form of assessment (congruence) perhaps it is not surprising that students also have difficulty in understanding the process, and often have unrealistic expectations of PLA (discord).

KEY LEARNING ACTIVITY 1

Obtain the following article: *Trowler, P. (1996) Angels in Marble? Accrediting Prior Experiential Learning in Higher Education. Studies in Higher Education. Vol. 21, No.1. p.17–30.*

Summarize possible biases in the APL process – you might want to organize these under the themes of *Cultural, Educational* or *Organizational*. Do you feel these biases are any different to those found within traditional forms of assessment?

In addition to the cultural, educational and organizational issues identified by Trowler (1996) there have also been some concerns regarding the clarity and transparency of the APL process. For example, an early article written by Paczuska and Randall (1996) stated:

> *... procedures are frequently informal, may be poorly documented, and implicit in admissions practice and in any credit awarded, rather than explicit. For the prospective student the process may be in accessible unless they happen to come into contact with a particular individual tutor. For tutors and guidance workers who advise prospective students the details are so often unclear.*
>
> *Paczuska and Randall (1996)*

A later study in the UK by Merrifield *et al.* (2000:3) indicated that although APL practice had been developing since the 1980s, it was still an area which was not well known or understood by students or academics.

In particular, Merrifield *et al.* indicated that mechanisms for APL were unwieldy, and were not user-friendly, nor were the potential benefits of APL well known to employers. The authors concluded that a gap between policy and practice existed.

More recently a study by the National Institute for Adult Continuing Education (NIACE) in 2008 also reported that PLA in Higher Education was still characterized by inconsistency and lack of coherence.

GUIDELINES FOR APL PRACTICE

Early attempts to lend clarity to the APL process emphasized the importance of guidelines and principles for APL practice. For example, in the USA the Council for Adult and Experiential Learning (CAEL) first devised the following guidelines:

- Credit should be awarded only for learning and not for experience.
- College credit should be awarded only for college-level learning.
- Credit should be awarded only for learning that has a balance, appropriate to the subject, between theory and practical application.
- The determination of competence levels and of credit awards must be made by appropriate subject matter and academic experts.
- Credit should be appropriate to the academic context in which it is accepted.
- Credit awards and their transcript entries should be monitored to avoid giving credit twice for the same learning.
- Policies and procedures applied to assessment, including provision for appeal, should be fully disclosed and prominently available.
- Fees charged for assessment should be based on the services performed in the process and not determined by the amount of credit awarded.
- All personnel involved in the assessment of learning should receive adequate training for the functions they perform, and there should be provision for their continued professional development.
- Assessment programmes should be regularly monitored, reviewed, evaluated, and revised as needed to reflect changes in the needs being served and in the state of the assessment arts.

Established in 1989, CAEL guidelines primarily addressed organizational issues for APL. However, the importance of these guidelines cannot be overstated for they have significantly influenced both policy and practice at an international level for many years.

Canada

Later, In 1997, the Canadian Labour Force Development Board (CLFDB) published the following minimum standards for PLAR:

- PLAR must be accessible and relevant to people as individuals. It must focus on the unique needs and abilities of the individual.
- Assessment and recognition must be of learning (knowledge and skills acquired through study or experience) not of experience.

- The PLAR process must be fair and equitable. It must be barrier-free and bias-free.
- The PLAR process must be efficient. It must make the best use of resources for the individual.
- The PLAR process must be effective. It must provide the opportunity for recognition of prior learning, but it must not hold out false promise.
- The PLAR process must be transparent. The individual must know the criteria and standards used to assess his or her skills and knowledge.
- The assessment must be reliable. The criteria and standards must be recognized and respected by all the labour market partners. This principle applies to occupational and skills standards, the learning outcomes stated for a specific course or training programme, and the credentials required for a specific job or occupational group.
- The assessment tools and their PLAR application must be recognized and accepted by all the labour market partners.
- Individuals assessing prior learning must be trained to perform this task.
- The assessing organization must provide a number of ways to carry out an assessment.
- Individuals should have the opportunity to choose how their assessment will be done. If necessary, they should get help to make their choice.
- Recognition awarded through PLAR should be considered equal to recognition awarded in the traditional manner.
- Recognition awarded through PLAR should be transferable between organizations, provinces and territories.
- PLAR must be an option or opportunity, not a mandatory process.
- If a person is not satisfied with the PLAR assessment, an appeal procedure must be available.

The influence of CAEL is apparent within these guidelines. However, the CLFDB only addressed organizational issues, with no real attempt to define or illuminate the role of the practitioner, the learner, or the APL process.

United Kingdom

In an attempt to clarify the role of the **APL practitioner,** the UK South East Education Consortium (**SEEC**) published their Code of Practice for APL in 1995. This included the following operational guidelines.

- Information about AP(E)L should be accessible to all applicants.
- Where academic staff are involved in the guidance and counselling of students in the preparation of AP(E)L evidence, they should not normally be the sole assessors of that evidence.
- The role and responsibilities of students will be made explicit in the AP(E)L process.
- Experience on its own is insufficient grounds for gaining credit. APEL credits the learning which the learner can evidence from prior experience.
- Evidence of learning must be assessed by academic staff using whatever means are appropriate.
- The AP(E)L process must be equitable and capable of scrutiny and enhance quality.
- Charges for AP(E)L, where they occur, and the criteria for these, should be clear to students and the institution.
- Where there is a maximum and/or minimum volume of credit allowed for AP(E)L, such limits should be made clear.

The above guidelines were revised in 2003 and again in 2005 to support the introduction of guidelines for APL devised by the QAA in 2004. The QAA guidelines were developed for faculties of higher education and currently offer principles and prompts for university staff undertaking prior learning assessment. However, the QAA (2004:13) state that their guidelines are not: '... a "how to do it manual" and do not provide models of practice or a detailed account of approaches and procedures to be followed'. The QAA guidelines an be found at: http://www.qaa.ac.uk/Publications/InformationAndGuidance/Pages/Guidelines-on-the-accreditation-of-prior-learning-September-2004.aspx.

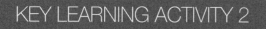

KEY LEARNING ACTIVITY 2

Obtain a copy of QAA guidelines for APL and compare these with your own organization's guidelines for APL practice.

1 Do the QAA guidelines explain the role of the APL practitioner in enough detail for you? What similarities or differences do you notice?

2 Discuss with your APL co-ordinator, or a respected colleague, how these similarities or differences might influence the role of the APL practitioner?

STANDARDS FOR APL PRACTICE

A good example of the development of standards for assessment practice is the work of the Training and Development Lead Body (1995) who first defined the competencies required of the vocational assessor through the process of *functional analysis*.

The TDLB standards (1995) outlined the key purpose, functions, activities and performance indicators relating to the work of assessors. The *key purpose* defined the function of *all* vocational assessors, including APL practitioners. The *function* described how the key purpose was to be achieved. The *activities* indicated how the key function was to be achieved. Finally, *Performance indicators* outlined the standard to be achieved during the process of assessment.

Therefore, according to the TDLB (1995) the key purpose of an assessor was to: *'review progress and to assess achievement, so that individuals and organizations can achieve their education and training objectives'.*

Also, according to the TDLB (1995) the functions and activities of Assessors were to:

1 Prepare the candidate for assessment. This includes the following activities:
   a) help the candidate to identify relevant learning;
   b) agree to and review an action plan for demonstration of prior learning; and
   c) help the candidate to prepare and present evidence for assessment.
2 Assess the candidate. This included the following activities:
   a) agree to and review an assessment plan;
   b) judge evidence and provide feedback; and
   c) make an assessment decision using differing sources of evidence and provide feedback.

The TDLB standards have been modified several times since they were first introduced in the UK. For example, they have been adapted from the original D32 and D33 standard and applied to the emergent A1 standard. Despite this, they remain an exemplar for best practice – as individuals who have completed a D32, D33 or A1 award are not required to undertake any further qualification before they work as a QCF assessor – rather they are only expected to attend an update.

Although the TDLB standards are regarded as an exemplar within the further education and vocational sectors, their use in Higher Education is highly controversial as many believe their use represents a mechanistic or behavioural view of learning , which (it is claimed) introduces the potential for social and political control; and is therefore a threat to the academic freedom that many universities within the UK enjoy (Day, 2012).

BENCHMARKS FOR APL PRACTICE

The Canadian Association for Prior Learning Assessment (**CAPLA**) have adapted the work of the TDLB (1995) and devised their own **benchmarks** for practice (see Chapter 4). This work has also been repeated in the UK (Day, 2011 and 2012).

Benchmarks for APL can be beneficial, for example, CAPLA conclude that benchmarking is: '... *a process that tends to build consensus and can be used in combination with other methods of job analysis*'. (Day, 2000a:124). CAPLA also confirm that:

> *... the process of benchmarking has a high degree of internal validity and it is sensitive to the qualities, characteristics and processes that help to define Practitioner behaviour.*

> *Day (2000b:124)*

Benchmarking is a continuous, systematic search for, and implementation of, best practices that may lead to improved performance. The goals of benchmarking are to build on the success of others, and to address **current** best practice. Benchmarking for is a beneficial process as it:

- *focuses on client needs* – this is fundamental to adult learning;
- *adapts industry-best practices* – best practice from education institutions;
- *helps to set relevant, realistic and achievable goals* – an open and transparent process for individuals and assessors; and
- *tests the quality of programme delivery* – students, employers and educational institutions must be able to see that the process is rigorous and credible.

The strengths, weaknesses, opportunities and potential threats of using benchmarks for APL are outlined by CAPLA (2000) – see Figure 1.4 below:

FIGURE 1.4   Strengths, weaknesses, opportunities and threats of benchmarks for APL

1   Strengths:
- Use of benchmarks will ensure that will become a defensible process.
- Provides a sense of reliability, equality and fairness.
- Improves accountability and transparency in the assessment process.
- Identifies what is possible, what is feasible, and what is acceptable.
- Ensures consistency of approach, particularly for workplace-based assessment.
- Will improve the rigor and fairness of the assessment process.
- Identifies the resources needed for assessment.
- Individuals will become more aware of requirements for assessment, thereby improving access to.
- Protects the rights of the learner.
- There will be more direction for faculty, thereby increasing confidence in the process.
- Provides a common understanding and communication between stakeholders.
- Identifies an ethical process for the professional.
- Improves mobility for the assessor.

2   Weaknesses
- Potential cultural or class bias.
- The language and standard adopted may be inappropriate.
- Danger of a '*cookie cutter approach*' i.e. one size fits all.
- There is a potential conflict of interest if a practitioner advises and assesses.
- Costly, will only happen if government funding is available or if employers can commit the resources.

3   Opportunities
- There is little information on available – practitioners will welcome the direction that benchmarks can provide.
- Can provide a methodology and/or a process for adult learning e.g. learning in the workplace; the promotion of client-centred approaches to learning.
- Can assist in the accreditation and articulation process between institutions.

FIGURE 1.4 **Strengths, weaknesses, opportunities and threats of benchmarks for APL (continued)**

- Can be used as a basis for training and certification; this will lead to credibility and acceptance of the assessor role.
- Benchmarks for may be transferable e.g. quality audit, workplace assessment, academic assessment.
- Can give credibility to what are traditionally known as '*soft*' skills e.g. employability skills by identifying a rigorous and consistent approach for assessment.
- Can motivate educational institutions to define curricula in outcomes-based language.

4   Potential Threats

- The individual or the Assessor may see benchmarks as unrealistic expectations.
- Benchmarks may re-define the role of the practitioner – a potential threat for faculty.
- Assessors will come under greater scrutiny, especially if there is an appeal.
- There may be a demand for '*perfection*' by the purchasers and commissioners of education.
- Universities may reject any prescriptive process or '*top down*' approaches to certification of Practitioners e.g. from government departments.
- Traditional values and beliefs about assessment may well generate resistance e.g. a credential is only valuable if few people possess it.
- Potential bureaucracy of assessment e.g. N/SVQs.
- Risk of reductionism i.e. there may be a 'whole' which is overlooked.

According to the CAPLA, the key purpose of the APL Assessor is to:

Review progress and/or assess achievements, so that individuals and organizations can achieve their personal development and/or education and training objectives.

CAPLA (2000)

The performance indicators relating to the key purpose and each of the functions and activities of the APL Practitioner will be examined in greater detail in Chapter 2.

SUMMARY

This introductory chapter has described the concept of APL and its relationship to adult learning theory. The potential benefits of APL to learners, employers and education institutions have been outlined and the principles which are fundamental to rigorous assessment of prior learning, and the establishment of a credit based system have also been discussed. The economic and social factors influencing the development of a credit based framework have been reviewed and emergent guidelines, standards and benchmarks for practice have been identified in an attempt to make the role of the APL practitioner much more explicit, and transparent.

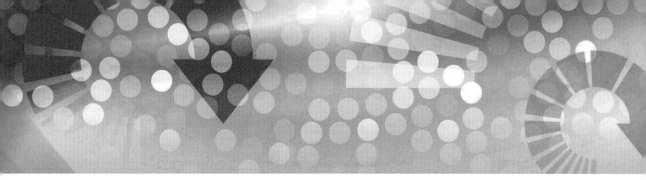

CHAPTER 2
BENCHMARKS FOR
ASSESSMENT OF
PRIOR LEARNING

Chapter 1 described the concept of APL and its theoretical underpinnings. It also outlined the potential bene-fits of APL, and the cultural, social and organizational factors currently influencing APL practice. Chapter 1 also discussed how emerging guidelines, standards and benchmarks are being used to resolve issues currently influencing APL practice.

This chapter will examine in more detail the role of the APL practitioner, drawing upon the original work of the Canadian Association for Prior Learning Assessment (Day, 2000b, 2001a and 2001b) and newly emerging benchmarks for practice in the UK to clarify the role of the APL advisor and assessor (Day, 2011).

At the end of this Chapter the reader will be able to:

● Outline the *key purpose, functions and activities* of the APL practitioner.

● Outline the functions and activities of the *APL Adviser, APL Assessor and APL Coordinator*.

● Identify key factors which might influence the role of the APL practitioner.

● Compare and contrast *direct* versus *indirect* evidence of prior learning.

An APL practitioner is an individual who utilizes learner-focused activities to formatively or summatively assess an individual's prior learning either for academic credit or recognition of occupational and/or professional competence. The key purpose of an APL Practitioner is to:

Review progress and/or assess achievements; so that individuals and organizations can achieve their personal development and/or education and training objectives. This includes assessment of individuals for academic credit and professional certification …

Day (2011:58)

This definition includes the work of the *APL adviser* who guides, assists and formatively assesses the learner – sometimes one-on-one, sometimes in small groups – in order to identify learning strengths and learning needs. It also includes the work of the *APL assessor* who summatively assesses individuals in order to award a final grade or to make a final decision about their competence.

APL assessors who summatively assess individuals should be competent and knowledgeable in the outcomes or competencies they are assessing. Within post-secondary education institutions the assessor is usually a subject-matter expert from faculty. In work place education and training programmes the assessor is usually an experienced member of staff who is occupationally or professionally competent and is trained in assessment skills.

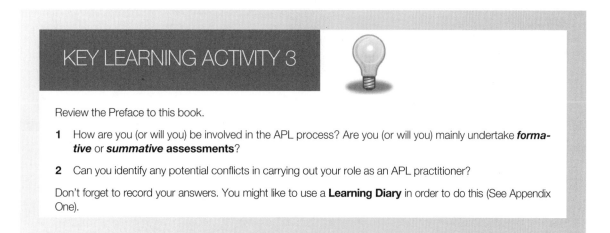

KEY LEARNING ACTIVITY 3

Review the Preface to this book.

1   How are you (or will you) be involved in the APL process? Are you (or will you) mainly undertake **formative** or **summative** assessments?

2   Can you identify any potential conflicts in carrying out your role as an APL practitioner?

Don't forget to record your answers. You might like to use a **Learning Diary** in order to do this (See Appendix One).

An APL *co-ordinator* may also be involved in the guidance and assessment of individuals, but will also be involved in maintaining, submitting and revising the use of assessment documents and records, for example, registration, orientation plans, assessment plans, assessment and certification procedures, appeals procedures. Also, providing advice and support to advisers and assessors, for example, initial training, trouble shooting, methods and resource development, continuing professional development and updating of assessors. The co-ordinator may also be involved in monitoring assessments and ensuring consistency in the assessment process, for example, establishment of sampling frameworks for the purpose of statistical analysis and report writing, conducting regular assessor meetings for the purpose of developing consistency in assessment processes, individual needs and equal opportunities monitoring.

ESTABLISHING THE APL PRACTITIONER ROLE

When establishing their role, APL practitioners should expect to encounter some initial tensions within their organizations. Such tensions may arise in the following situations. *Firstly*, between work colleagues who might question the rationale for selecting one person as a adviser or assessor, rather than another. *Secondly*, between APL assessor and manager, when the assessor negotiates time and space out of normal work activities in order to undertake assessments. *Thirdly*, within individual APL assessors, particularly when they realize that they will be held accountable for their assessment decisions. *Fourthly*, when individuals realize the need to reconcile the demands of being an APL assessor with the demands of being an APL adviser, so that objectivity can be maintained and any potential conflict of interest between the two roles can be avoided or minimized.

The APL practitioner's role demands a range of interactions with individuals from within and outside the organization. Interactions with adult learners include: pre-assessment guidance and action planning; observation and ongoing collaboration; providing feedback on performance and or competence.

In addition, APL practitioners may be required to: meet with their peers for the purpose of developing consistency in the application of assessment methods; meet with others in order to justify their assessment decisions, for example, APL advisers, APL co-ordinators, heads of faculty, heads of human resource development, external advisers, etc.; and liase with adult learners, managers, administrators and faculty to report on individual progress and to comment on resources for APL.

It is essential that regular contact is maintained with faculty, other APL advisers and assessors, as well as the APL co-ordinator so that competence in assessment and the integrity of the process is maintained. In order to competently carry out their duties, practitioners need to have a clear understanding of the process and how it relates to their role. They also need to have an appreciation of the competencies required of the adviser and the assessor (See Appendix One).

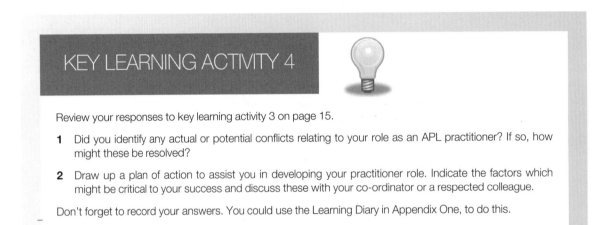

KEY LEARNING ACTIVITY 4

Review your responses to key learning activity 3 on page 15.

1 Did you identify any actual or potential conflicts relating to your role as an APL practitioner? If so, how might these be resolved?

2 Draw up a plan of action to assist you in developing your practitioner role. Indicate the factors which might be critical to your success and discuss these with your co-ordinator or a respected colleague.

Don't forget to record your answers. You could use the Learning Diary in Appendix One, to do this.

At some point in their development, Practitioners may need to demonstrate that they are competent in the relevant activities and functions outlined in the final learning activity, Chapter Seven. For example, what are the specific competencies which support the work of the adviser? These competencies are slightly different than those required of the assessor. The difference depends upon whether one is involved in formative or summative assessment. For example, the APL assessor will often make a final appraisal of an individual's work in order that academic credit can be awarded or competence confirmed. Whereas the APL adviser is more often involved in informal or ongoing developmental work. The APL assessor carries out the following activities:

- agreeing to and reviewing an assessment plan;
- judging evidence and providing feedback; and
- making an assessment decision and giving feedback.

Whereas the APL adviser mainly carries out the following activities:

- helping the individual to identify relevant learning;
- agreeing to and reviewing an action plan for demonstration of prior learning;
- and helping the individual to prepare and present evidence for assessment.

Some activities are performed by both the adviser and the assessor. For example, both of these practitioners are involved in action planning, making an appropriate judgement about evidence, and providing feedback to adult learners.

KEY LEARNING ACTIVITY 5

Compare your current (or intended role) as a practitioner with the functions and activities outlined on the previous page.

1 Would you say that you are (or will be) an APL Adviser, or an APL Assessor, or both?

2 What activities (if any) differentiate the role of adviser and assessor within your organization?

3 Within your organization what activities do the adviser and assessor have in common?

Record your answers in your Learning Diary (See Appendix One).

Many APL practitioners now undertake both the role of the advisor *and* the role of the assessor – as part of a team-based approach to assessment. Many assessment skills are common to both the adviser and the assessor roles. Each of the activities relating to the role of the assessor and the adviser are now outlined.

The role of the APL assessor

1. Agreeing to and reviewing an assessment plan

Assessors may be involved in planning the most appropriate time, place and method for an individual's assessment. There is no prescribed format for this but they will need to take into account and discuss:

- the outcome or competence to be assessed;
- an appropriate time and place for the assessment;
- the type of evidence that needs to be gathered e.g. how will competence be assessed as well as supporting knowledge and understanding;
- any aspects of confidentiality that may apply;
- any ethical implications for assessment e.g. how will the safety of a third party be maintained;
- any special assessment requirements – the individual may be a shift worker, nervous, or use English or French as a second language; and
- the assessor and the adult learner need to make sure that they agree with the plan and that this agreement is appropriately recorded.

An Example of an assessment plan is given on the next page.

2. Judging evidence and providing feedback

Practitioners may be involved in formatively or summatively reviewing the performance and/or competence of individuals, and evaluating them against the criteria for the competencies or outcomes being assessed. These outcomes or competencies should be made available to both the Practitioner and the adult learner before an assessment is made of the learner's competence.

Practitioners are often required to review tasks and activities associated with the adult learner's field of study, place of work or chosen profession. This may be difficult to substantiate without the use of checklists or assessment records, which should be signed by the practitioner and the adult learner. To help validate an assessment decision it is often useful to refer to examples of products that have arisen from the learner's work/studies. These products should be relevant to the criteria being assessed.

Practitioners will often need to ask questions in order to explore the supporting knowledge and understanding relating to the criteria which is being assessed. It is important not to lead the individual; i.e. that the question does not suggest the answer.

Questions could be *spontaneous*: verbal questions arising naturally from the evidence being reviewed. It is advisable to jot them down, along with the adult learner's response – as far as is reasonably possible i.e. do not let this distract from the work at hand.

EXAMPLE ASSESSMENT PLAN

Learner:	Fred Smith	**Adult Learner Identification No.**	00001
Organization:	Peabody International	**APL Adviser/Assessor:**	Malcolm Day
Outcomes/Competencies:		**Criteria:**	Unit One H&S 1a, 1b. 1c.

Peabody 's Workplace Development programme
Health and Safety at Work, Unit One

1. Assessment opportunities:
Fred is the workplace health and safety officer with responsibility for attending workplace accidents and administering first aid. He is also responsible for training other workers in first aid procedure. Evidence of Fred's competence can be provided by **letters of validation** *from those whom he has assisted, plus records of incidents he has maintained (with client's permission). Fred always evaluates his training sessions; these evaluations are available in written form.*

2. Assessment methods:
Letter of validation: three validation letters from clients Fred has assisted.
Workplace Product: copies of Fred's incident reports relating to the above.
Workplace product: copy of evaluation forms from at least three training sessions Fred has conducted.
Interview/oral questioning: discuss the contents of Fred's portfolio and how these relate to criteria Unit One.

3. Resources required:
Blank letter of validation × three
Copy portfolio development guidelines

4. Action to be taken by Assessor/Adviser:
Malcolm to provide Fred with blank copies of letter of validation, plus portfolio guidelines.
Malcolm to arrange interview to discuss Fred's portfolio and how it relates to criteria 1a. 1b. 1c.

5. Action to be taken by the Learner:
Fred to compile a portfolio to include letters of validation, copy of incident records and copies of evaluation forms from training sessions.
Fred to get written permission from clients/administrators to use incident records.
Fred to let Malcolm have diary dates for meeting re: discussion of portfolio.

Signature of Adviser/Assessor: _____ Date: _____
Signature of Learner: _____ Date: _____

Questions could be *pre-planned*: a series of written questions necessary to ask of the individual, which are prepared in advance. APL practitioners and their colleagues could develop a question bank. This has the advantage that other assessors have checked the questions to ensure they directly relate to the criteria being assessed. These questions are confidential and should not be disclosed to individuals prior to the assessment.

Questions could be *spontaneous and pre-planned*: as one becomes more familiar with the required criteria and more experienced in the art of interviewing, it may be possible to combine both strategies in order to get a greater appreciation of the individual's performance/competence and underpinning knowledge and understanding. Questions should cover *processes*, as well as *outcomes*. It is important to pay particular attention to situations which have not been verified by others.

Individuals can become extremely nervous when subjected to questioning. Questions are best kept simple and should be directly related to the criteria being assessed. A quiet room is needed, free from interruptions and distractions. Also, it is helpful to have a list of relevant questions on a separate sheet of paper to which to refer. The sheet of paper should also have a blank column in which to record the individual's answers. It is important to sign and date it and to get the adult learner's signature as well.

3. Asking questions

When asking questions it is important to remember that learners have to first hear what is being said, then understand the question, think about it, search their memory, formulate an answer, then give the answer – this takes time. Remember to:

- ask questions in an interested manner and with a natural tone of voice;
- word questions in simple and straightforward language – avoid textbook jargon;
- pace the conversation and allow some time before going to the next question;
- ask questions which require more than a yes/no response;
- ask questions which only directly relate to the criteria being assessed;
- pose questions which do not suggest the answer; and
- encourage the learner to give a full and complete answer.

Also, try to avoid:

- ambiguous questions;
- trick questions;
- repeating the learner's answer;
- sarcasm at the wrong answers;
- asking mainly factual questions;
- repeating the question, it's probably better to rephrase it;
- asking questions just to prolong the assessment;
- asking questions that the learner will not be able to answer; and
- putting unnecessary pressure on the learner.

4. Making an assessment decision and giving feedback

Once the evidence has been collected, the practitioner has to decide whether the individual has met the required criteria and inform him or her of the decision. Similarly if competencies or outcomes have not been met, the individual needs to be informed in a positive and constructive way, how this gap can be filled. It is important to be clear and concise about this – in fact it is helpful to record this information for the person.

When giving personal feedback to the adult learner it is important to be as sensitive as possible. Any negative comments may be harmful. It is also important to give the individual one's undivided attention and to respond appropriately to how he or she may be feeling after the assessment. The discussion can be initiated by asking how the individual thought the assessment went – this will help open up the feedback process and encourage him or her to share any concerns without fear of criticism. Individuals often identify gaps that have become obvious during the assessment process enabling the Practitioner to build upon their strengths and work toward the development of a realistic plan to help overcome any shortfalls. It will take time to carry this out effectively. A quiet room, free from interruptions should help. However, it is one's personal approach, the way in which interest and concern are expressed, that will help to ensure a successful outcome to this process.

THE INTERVIEW

Interviews are an essential ingredient in the process. They provide both the adult learner and the assessor with an excellent opportunity to seek additional information, ask for clarification and engage in dialogue aimed at building on learner strengths and exploring realistic alternatives if additional learning/evidence is needed. Skilled interviewers pay close attention to both verbal and non-verbal cues during the interview and respond appropriately to them. During the interview it is important to pay particular attention to the following factors which can have a significant impact on the outcomes of the interview.

- *posture* – relaxed, upright, facing person at a reasonable distance.
- *gestures* – balanced, open, relaxed and non-threatening.
- *facial expression* – firm and pleasant.
- *eye contact* – gentle, direct, relaxed gaze, same eye level.
- *voice, tone and volume* – low-pitched, medium volume, gentle.
- *language* – honest, open and to the point, giving praise and honest feedback. sharing and taking responsibility for your own feelings.
- *timing* – putting your own point of view across and encouraging the learner to do the same.

Remember to clearly and accurately record the agreed-upon outcomes of the interview, identifying how any shortfalls can be overcome, the support the learner will need to overcome them and any agreed upon timelines. An example of an assessment record is given below.

SAMPLE ASSESSMENT RECORD

Learner: Fred Smith   **Adult Learner Identification No.**   00001
Organization: Peabody International   **APL Adviser/Assessor:**   Malcolm Day
Outcomes/Competencies: **Criteria:**   Unit One H&S 1a, 1b. 1c.
Peabody's Workplace Development programme
Health and Safety at Work, Unit One

Evidence methods used:
Discussion regarding Fred's role as a certified workplace health and safety officer, against criteria for H&S 1a, 1b and 1c (see portfolio) including administrative tasks and training role. A copy of the questions I asked are attached.

   Three different letters of validation from those whom Fred has assisted (see portfolio) e.g. a client who fainted, a client who cut her hand and a client who suffered a heart attack.

   Copies of evaluation sheets from three different training sessions Fred has conducted e.g. Principles of First Aid, CPR and fractures and sprains.

Areas where competence/outcomes have been achieved:
Fred has demonstrated that he is competent in all of the activities outlined in H&S Unit 1a, 1b, 1c.

Areas where competence/outcomes have not yet been achieved:
Fred is now collecting evidence relating to the Advanced First Aid at Work Module.

Assessor's comments (continue on back of sheet if you wish).
Responses to my questions (attached) and comprehensive workplace documentation placed in Fred's portfolio indicates that he is more than competent in the criteria required. Well done Fred!

Learner's comments (continue on back of sheet if you wish).
I was given very clear guidelines on how to collect evidence against the criteria required. This made the compilation of the portfolio much easier.

Signature of Adviser/Assessor: _____   Date: _____
Signature of Learner: _____   Date: _____

The role of the APL adviser

1. Helping the individual to identify relevant learning

The advise works with individuals and groups to help them identify relevant prior learning. It is possible to collect many forms of evidence to demonstrate prior learning. This section will concentrate on what is meant by *sufficient* evidence in relation to the use of a:

- Learning diary
- Letter of validation
- Simulation

2. Learning diary

A learning diary can provide evidence that learners have the necessary supporting knowledge and understanding relating to an outcome or competence. When completed, the learning diary can be submitted to the Assessor, who will then ask questions about it. For example, whether it is the learner's own work, how it relates to the criteria being assessed, as well as questions about the content of the material.

In keeping a learning diary, the learner will need to identify a strategy that will demonstrate he or she has the appropriate knowledge relating to the criteria being assessed. For example, he or she may need to search out new and relevant information, read it, appraise it and record it in a meaningful way. The learner may also want to have a discussion with a more experienced colleague or mentor, or wish to attend a professional development activity or study day.

The learner will also need identify what he or she has learned, taking into account any reading, professional development activities and/or any discussions with others; then apply what he or she has learned to his or her practice by indicating how any new knowledge will be used in the workplace to solve a problem or deal with a contingency.

Finally the learner will identify the evidence he or she can use to demonstrate appropriate knowledge. This will need to be discussed with the assessor and it may include a bibliography, any notes taken, copies of any diagrams produced, any certificates received, etc.

An example of a learning diary and how it might be completed is provided below.

SAMPLE LEARNING DIARY

Your Name: _____   **Your Identification No.** _____
Organization: _____   **Your Adviser is:** _____

1. What is my strategy for learning?
After examining the criteria to be achieved, you could seek relevant information at the library or have a discussion with a colleague at work or with a mentor. Keep a record of what you do as this could count as part of the evidence you present in your portfolio.

2. What have I learned?
Based on the information you gained from the above activities, you will need to identify the knowledge you have gained, and indicate how it relates to the criteria to be assessed.

3. How will I apply this knowledge?
State how the knowledge gained will be applied to your field of study or occupation. For example, you may use it to solve an existing problem or you could describe how it might be used to solve a potential problem.

4. What evidence can I demonstrate?
List the possible sources of evidence which demonstrate you have the appropriate knowledge for each of the criteria against which you are being assessed. For example; a record of the reading you have undertaken, a copy of any notes you have made, any certificates of attendance you have obtained at training sessions. Don't forget to make a copy of any learning diaries you have completed in your portfolio!

5. Adviser comments
The APL Adviser will need to record whether he/she agrees that you have the necessary supporting knowledge, and understanding and confirm the outcomes or competencies to which this relates. The Adviser will do this by counter-signing this form and making any appropriate comments. These records should be recorded in your portfolio.

Your Signature: _____   Date: _____
Signature of Adviser: _____   Date: _____

3. Validation letters

Validation letters can provide an indirect and authenticated account of the adult learner's performance/competence. They may be collected from colleagues, supervisors, managers, customers, suppliers, etc. Letters of validation should:

- be specific to an activity or product;
- give a brief description of the circumstances and context of the observation;
- give a brief description of the background and qualifications of the signatory;
- give a brief background to the observed activity; and
- identify aspects of the outcome or competence demonstrated and how it relates to the set criteria.

It is helpful to provide a checklist to the individual writing the validation letter, the signatory, to link the learner's performance/competence directly to the appropriate outcome or competency.

The signatory may simply authenticate a piece of work as having been produced by the learner. In other cases, the signatory may provide an account of the learner's performance and comment on it in relation to the appropriate outcome or competency. It is important that signatories are familiar with the set criteria and are able to comment authoritatively on the learner's performance/competence. Before accepting evidence from a letter of validation, the adviser will need to:

- judge the authenticity and validity of the evidence;
- check that the evidence is clear about the standards being covered; and
- check that the signatory can be contacted for authentication of the validation letter, if necessary

An example of a letter of validation is provided below.

SAMPLE VALIDATION LETTER

Learner's Name: Fred Smith   **Learner's Identification Number:** 00001

1. Declaration:

I have read and understood the outcomes/competencies required and I am able to state that the above individual can meet the following requirements:

Competence/Outcomes: Health and Safety Unit One

_____

Competencies/Criteria: 1a, 1b and 1c

_____

_____

2. Evidence to support the above statement i.e. I am able to state this because . . .

Fred looked after me when I cut my hand at work. He laid me flat, raised my hand in the air and applied a firm bandage to control the bleeding. He covered me with a blanket and told me not to eat or drink anything and then arranged an ambulance to get me to hospital. When I returned to work the next day, Fred helped me fill out the accident report book. Fred was calm throughout the incident and I really felt safe and reassured by him.

3. Details of person signing the Letter of Validation

Name: Joan Smith   Designation: Shop floor worker
Qualifications: Body Shop Operative   Telephone: Extension 242
Relationship of Witness to Learner: Client: E-mail:
Address: The Body Shop, Peabody International _____   Telephone Number: Ext. 242

Your Signature: _____   Date: _____
Signature of Adviser: _____   Date: _____

NB: You may be contacted by an APL Assessor to confirm your observations/comments.

4. Use of simulations

Any source of performance evidence other than the learner's normal, naturally-occurring work activity can be thought of as a simulation. However, before the learner decides to use simulation, all other sources of evidence should be examined to ensure that simulation is the most cost-effective and appropriate method.

Care must be taken to ensure that any simulated assessment meets the full requirements of the outcomes or competencies being assessed. The adviser must be confident that any competence demonstrated during the simulation can be transferred to the work environment and is therefore a realistic representation of the knowledge and performance/competence required.

Simulation could be used when there are issues relating to confidentiality and safety or to increase access to assessment. Some examples are given below:

- future requirements such as new technologies and work practices at the individual's workplace that do not offer opportunities to provide appropriate evidence;
- infrequent events such as an annual inventory or the outcome of a five-year business plan if waiting for the event to occur could delay assessment;
- avoiding risks to the individual or others in the work environment, e.g. cleaning procedures in cases of chemical contamination;
- procedures which may have complicated or dangerous consequences, e.g. testing for and repairing a gas leak;
- life-threatening conditions, such as resuscitation of a person who has stopped breathing; and
- situations in which collecting evidence would intrude on personal privacy or confidentiality.

Simulations allow the learner to develop and practice skills in a safe environment and can provide useful opportunities for developmental assessment and feedback. However, when simulations are used for assessing competence against a standard they must be set up to reflect real activities and conditions. All simulations must provide for valid and reliable assessment of the required outcomes and criteria.

When planning to use simulation, the adviser and the learner should consider the following questions:

- what arrangements have been made for identifying sources of evidence? e.g. workplace, work cement simulation at the evidence planning stage?
- when workplace evidence is not available, have opportunities to use work cements and job rotation been fully explored?
- do other faculty/staff or assessors share a common understanding of simulation?
- what systems, processes and design criteria are in place to support the development and design of simulations?
- are the simulations cost-effective when compared to other methods of generating and gathering evidence?
- what arrangements have been made for briefing those who are to be assessed through simulation?

5. Agreeing to and reviewing an action plan for demonstration of prior learning

Learners might think that they already have the necessary knowledge and experience required to demonstrate that they can meet some of the outcomes or competencies of a programme. Much of the evidence that can be used for this has already been discussed and includes certificates and transcripts, from previous courses; work records and products; and letters of validation.

Some organizations keep a comprehensive account of staff training activities and they regularly carry out staff performance reviews. Other organizations issue workers with a personal handbook which records comments from supervisors on their performance at work. The outcomes of these staff development activities may be used as evidence, provided they relate to the criteria being assessed and they can be substantiated.

Learners may find that they can organize evidence to demonstrate several outcomes or competencies at the same time. If the assessment process is to be meaningful, it is important to consider the possibility of using this whole or 'holistic' approach to APL – rather than reducing the process to a series of unconnected observations and tasks. In doing this advisers will find that:

- the process will become more interesting;
- evidence will become more meaningful and efficient;

- it will avoid unnecessary repetition;
- use of learners' achievements will be maximized; and
- it will save valuable time and energy which can be applied elsewhere.

Learners will need to take into account the way in which they organize their work and/or learning in order to make best use of the evidence they are generating. One way of doing this is to build up a portfolio of learning and experience. This process can be initiated by undertaking a self-assessment of one's current skills, abilities and competencies. The results of this activity and any supporting evidence can be included in a portfolio.

6. Help the individual to prepare and present evidence for assessment

Evidence of prior learning can be collected in a portfolio. A portfolio is a record kept in a binder, a file or a folder – of an individual's prior learning achievements – what she or he knows and can do. Some portfolios are extremely comprehensive and wide-ranging, some are more narrowly and specifically focused – depending on the purposes, objectives and goals of the learner.

SUMMARY

This Chapter has examined in detail the role of the APL practitioner, drawing upon the original work of the Canadian Association for Prior Learning Assessment, and newly emerging benchmarks for UK practice to clarify the role of the APL advisor and assessor. The *key purpose, functions and activities* of the *APL practitioner have been outlined* and the *factors which might influence the APL practitioner role* have been discussed. Finally, the use of *direct* versus *indirect* evidence of prior learning has been discussed, using a portfolio approach. While portfolios often contain many of the elements and components outlined within this Chapter, there is no single 'right' way to organize and present a portfolio. In fact, people often exercise a great deal of creativity in this regard.

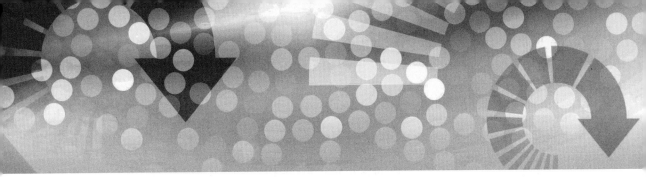

CHAPTER 3
DEVELOPMENTS IN THE UK – THE CASE OF PRE-REGISTRATION NURSING

This chapter focuses on the use of Assessment of Prior Learning (APL) within nurse education in the United Kingdom (UK). Nursing as a subject has a long-standing tradition of APL within post registration studies in the UK. More recently it has been considered for pre-registration curricula; prior learning in the form of experience and certificated learning with academic credit. Both can be used to demonstrate achievement of professional requirements but there must be opportunities available for this purpose:

Programme providers must have rigorous processes for accrediting both theory and practice learning.
NMC (2010a:57)

This chapter draws upon the definitions in Chapters 1 and 2 to explore the history of APL in nursing and post registration studies. The ramifications of moving nurse education into higher education and the emergence of new curricula which explicitly invite assessment and accreditation of prior learning for pre-registration nursing will be discussed. Academic institutions have rules about how much APL can contribute to an academic award. Where does this leave schools and faculties who are attempting to embrace generous APL guidance advocated by the professional regulatory and statutory body, the Nursing & Midwifery Council? The text explores some ideas and tensions.

At the end of this Chapter the reader will be able to:

- Describe how APL has been used within post registration study for nurses.

- Identify the circumstances for applying APL within pre-registration nursing curricula.

- Outline how APL can be recognized and accredited to comply with NMC guidance.

- Compare and contrast models and processes for APL within pre-registration nursing curricula.

NURSING AND APL

By the mid 1990s, nurse education in the UK had moved wholesale into the higher education sector. This was in response to the United Kingdom Central Council for Nursing, Midwifery and Health Visiting (UKCC) 1986 report *Project 2000: A new preparation for practice*. A nursing student would be expected to study to diploma level and be a '*knowledgeable doer*' (UKCC, 1986: 40). Diploma level is part of the Framework for Higher Education Qualifications in England, Wales and Northern Ireland (QAA, 2008), and comparable to the first two years of an undergraduate programme of study in terms of academic achievement. In reality nursing students usually undertook the course over three years to comply with professional regulatory requirements for the number of theory and practice hours completed. This is necessary for professional registration and to comply with European Union agreements. It is currently no less than 4600 hours, 2300 hours of which should be devoted to theory and 2300 hours in practice (NMC, 2010a: 8, 9)

Within ten years of the UKCC (1986) report it was clear courses leading to professional registration were not producing nurses *fit for purpose*. The UKCC, which was the professional regulatory and statutory body at the time and predecessor of the Nursing & Midwifery Council (NMC), set up the Commission for Education in 1998 led by Sir Leonard Peach. It coincided with an overhaul of the National Health Service (NHS) following a change of UK government. The Commission concluded in 1999 with the report *Fitness for Practice* (UKCC, 1999). Meanwhile, the new Labour government had produced their own ideas on where nursing, midwifery and health visiting should strengthen the underpinning values to meet the needs of the modern NHS. The *Making a Difference* publication included a new model for education and changes to the commissioning process for student places, (Department of Health, (DH) 1999). Lord (2002) and Kenny (2004) provide useful commentaries on the impact of *Fitness for Practice* (UKCC, 1999) and associated changes for nurse education policy. Kenny (2004) observed that nurse educators were marginalized at the time.

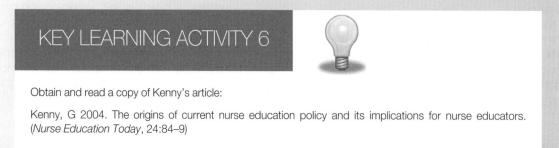

KEY LEARNING ACTIVITY 6

Obtain and read a copy of Kenny's article:

Kenny, G 2004. The origins of current nurse education policy and its implications for nurse educators. (*Nurse Education Today*, 24:84–9)

(continued)

- Consider the similarities and differences with nurse education in the current climate, in particular the relationship between higher education and service providers.
- Does the 'society-centred model' (p. 87) have any implications for future applicants?
- What about nurses who qualified with a diploma from this change in policy? How easy is it for them to become graduates today?

One of Sir Leonard Peach's recommendations (UKCC, 1999) was the use of APL within pre-registration nursing courses. This was to be encouraged in the first year or 'common foundation' of the programme to enable greater flexibility and recognition that applicants of varying ages and backgrounds bring important and relevant experience. Some applicants had not achieved the five General Certificate of Secondary Education (GCSEs) or equivalent that was typical of the minimum entry requirement for diploma courses at the time. The GSCEs normally had to include English, Maths and a science with at least C grade passes. See Ofqual (2009) for an explanation of these qualifications and the grades awarded. Instead, these individuals had undertaken National Vocational Qualifications (NVQs) in Care or Access to Further Education or Higher Education courses. The latter is a recognized diploma course to help prepare students for study in higher education.

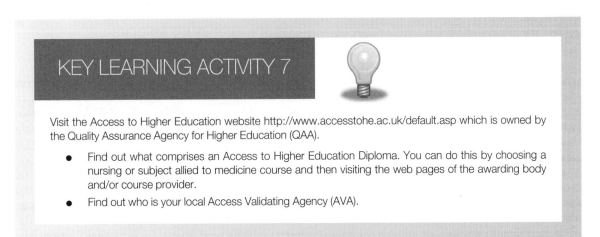

KEY LEARNING ACTIVITY 7

Visit the Access to Higher Education website http://www.accesstohe.ac.uk/default.asp which is owned by the Quality Assurance Agency for Higher Education (QAA).

- Find out what comprises an Access to Higher Education Diploma. You can do this by choosing a nursing or subject allied to medicine course and then visiting the web pages of the awarding body and/or course provider.
- Find out who is your local Access Validating Agency (AVA).

The QAA regulate the national recognition of Access to HE courses in England, Wales and Northern Ireland. These courses can now be used to meet the entry criteria for pre-registration nursing but in the late 1990s and into the new millennium were sometimes used to advance a student on a course with some recognition of academic credit previously achieved. Day (2013) refers to this practice earlier in this text. Similar applied to applicants with an NVQ in Care at Level 3 of the Qualifications and Curriculum Framework (QCF) (Lombardi *et al.*, 2004) and for those who already held a degree in a health-related subject. Flexibility was the key with '*stepping on*' and '*stepping off*' points, (DH, 1999:25). A School or faculty consequently had a very broad range of nursing students commencing the post 1999 *Making a Difference* curriculum. This was the revised curriculum in light of the Commission for Education (UKCC, 1999) and DH (1999) publications and became known as the MAD curriculum, (Lord, 2002).

Alongside the larger diploma programmes a number of schools and faculties also ran a pre-registration nursing degree. Still requiring professional regulatory and statutory body (NMC) approval these conjointly validated courses could also accommodate APL within the first year of the programme. The QAA (2001) produced degree benchmark statements for nursing to illustrate subject specific requirements as part of a larger framework for health professions. The three generic areas common to a number of professions allied to medicine are:

A Expectations of the health professional in providing patient/client services.

B The application of practice in securing, maintaining or improving health and well-being.

C Knowledge, understanding and skills that underpin the education and training of health care professionals.

Any review of these benchmarks, written more than ten years ago, will be influenced by the Bologna Process and its main objective of a European Higher Education Area (QAA, 2012). This encourages greater transparency of European education systems and facilitates student transfers across countries. The work of the professional, statutory and regulatory bodies (PSRBs) including the NMC will also impact on any revision. See *Professional, statutory and regulatory bodies; an explanation of their engagement with higher education* from the Higher Education Better Regulation Group (2011) to gain a greater insight into the role of PSRBs in course approval and quality assurance monitoring.

To explore the use of APL in undergraduate programmes leading to nurse registration it is useful to think first about APL for continuing professional development. Much can be learned from the processes and models that have been used for nurses undertaking post registration studies as a consequence of the Project 2000 and MAD curricula.

APL AND POST REGISTRATION STUDY FOR NURSES

Flexibility and broadening the entry gate have always been a priority for higher education. Johnson (2002) remarked that APL was one way of addressing this agenda in the 1980s when demographic patterns suggested there would be less traditional higher education applicants. He argued it could continue to attract different candidates who bring a wealth of experiential learning to their studies. '*Widening participation*' (WP) as it is now more commonly known is a key strand of government policy and evident within the reform plans for higher education in the UK, (Department for Business, Innovation and Skills, 2011: Chapter 5).

In nursing, widening participation has been important for continuing professional education. Following the implementation of Project 2000 (UKCC, 1986) qualified nurses worried they would get left behind and lose out on job opportunities to the new style nurse with a diploma. Could a qualified nurse, for example, mentor and assess a student if they had not studied to diploma level themselves? There was a need to develop flexible post registration courses for qualified nurses to achieve at least a diploma qualification. The NMC's decision to move all pre-registration nursing education to degree level by September 2013 (NMC, 2010b) has made this all the more pressing for those who have not studied within higher education. Qualified nurses do not present with traditional pre-requisites in the form of UCAS points as invited by the Universities and College Admissions Services (UCAS) for undergraduate courses. They mostly present with experience. Some will not have achieved diploma level studies because they qualified as a nurse before Project 2000 or had a career break and are now returning to employment. Others will have a diploma qualification and are looking to become a graduate if they are to succeed in the current healthcare environment and career structure defined by Agenda for Change and the Knowledge and Skills Framework (KSF), (DH, 2004a and b).

KEY LEARNING ACTIVITY 8

Agenda for Change and the career structure for nursing can be complex for those not familiar with the UK system.

- Visit the Flying Start NHS England website http://www.flyingstartengland.nhs.uk/ to gain an insight into what is required of newly registered nurses and the guidance offered.

- Look at the last part of the learning programme menu entitled *Career Pathways* to find information on the KSF and levels of the framework. Newly qualified practitioners registering with a PSRB (professional, statutory and regulatory body) usually commence employment at level 5 or Band 5 within the pay system of Agenda for Change.

- The NMC also have requirements for ongoing professional development. This is contained within the post registration education and practice (PREP) handbook (NMC, 2011b) and can be downloaded from the NMC website http://www.nmc-uk.org/Documents/Standards/NMC_Prep-handbook_2011.pdf.

As Project 2000 and subsequently the MAD curriculum were implemented qualified nurses began to study modules of credit in higher education institutions (HEI). Day (2013) explains the notion of a module or unit of learning earlier in this text. Modules normally belong to flexible pathways forming part of a diploma or degree course. For health care practitioners these are often commissioned for continuing professional education. Funding has tended to come from employers who have a vested interest in the design and composition of the courses; to provide education for nursing staff and others to deliver evidence-based care in clinical practice. Module credit accumulates for the academic qualification and can be transferred between HEIs. This takes place in the author's own institution under a local memorandum of agreement between three other HEIs and is useful for recognition of discrete NMC approved modules, for example, mentor preparation to meet NMC (2008) professional standards. It is also useful for when it is impractical or not cost-effective to offer the same provision in all HEIs because expertise, clinical experience or student numbers are not sufficient.

Depending on work pressures, funding and personal circumstances, currency of credit was sometimes an issue for qualified nurses seeking a diploma or a degree. Module credit would 'go out of date' although up to five years since achievement is normally acceptable and considered 'live credit'. APL became popular as a way of speeding up progress and reducing the cost. Johnson (2002) and Scott (2010) both remark on these aspects. Credit was usually the 'general' type where the APL candidate was seeking to fill credit gaps at an academic level. Sometimes it was 'specific', for example, the experience of having used the knowledge and skills of an older style mentor qualification. The qualification may not have carried credit and so referencing or mapping to the current professional standards (NMC 2008) with an explanatory narrative to demonstrate achievement, will attract specific credit that is equivalent to a conventional mentor preparation module with associated learning outcomes. In the UK, a mentor is someone who has undertaken a mentor preparation programme approved by the NMC in order to supervise and assess students leading to professional registration. Mentors are expected to attend annual updates to ensure they:

- Have current knowledge of NMC approved programmes.
- Are able to discuss the implications of changes to NMC requirements.
- Have an opportunity to discuss issues related to mentoring, assessment of competence and fitness for safe and effective practice.

NMC (2008:30)

Experiential learning from mentoring is therefore useful for claiming academic credit and the professional standards acknowledge the role of APL for this purpose, (NMC, 2008).

APL PROCESS

APL submissions at the author's institution are mostly for assessment of experiential learning. Increasingly, learning is derived from discrete events in the workplace such as study days, conferences and in-house courses, for example, Caddye and Hatfield (2011). The approach is learner-focused and *'developmental'* as described by Butterworth (1992 cited by Day, 2012 and Pokorny, 2012). The emphasis is on developing a reflective narrative to reveal the learning that has taken place as a result of the experience. Day (2013) mentions earlier in this text how this sits better with a pedagogy for higher education. Pokorny's (2012) small interpretative study attempted to take this further and look at the 'meaning making' from the perspective of both the APL practitioner and candidate using methodology from the academic literacies field. Empowering the candidate by adopting a transformative approach and negotiation of 'meaning making' requires *dialogic mediation* (Gravett and Henning (1998) cited by Pokorny, 2012). Knowledge is jointly constructed by the learner and the teacher. The learner is active in the co-construction and the teacher acts as a mediator. The relationship is one of mutual respect and learner-centred, all characteristics of adult learning theory, (Knowles, Holton and Swanson, 2011).

At the School of Nursing & Midwifery at the University of Brighton APL candidates attend an initial briefing workshop to learn about the APL process and its relevance to their intended course of study. If they wish to proceed and claim credit for their experiential learning they enrol on one of the APL modules. The briefing workshop and the module enrolment incur flat rate charges. An APL module has a broad aim and some generic learning outcomes set at an academic level (level 4, 5 or 6) and volume of credit, for example, 10, 20 or 30 credits. See QAA (2008) for further explanation of level and credit ratings. The APL candidate then negotiates an individual learning agreement with a member of academic staff who is an *'educational adviser'* (APL practitioner). The candidate selects the adviser based on subject expertise or geographical location to enable face to face advice if desired. The agreement includes personalized learning outcomes and negotiation of assessment methods.

Candidates often select a form of reflective narrative such as a case study or critical incident but assessment of clinical skills in practice by a mentor, or by simulation, are options within a flexible menu of assessment methods. The narratives are developed through discussion and formative feedback from the adviser, and then submitted at a negotiated summative assessment point as part of a portfolio of evidence. The summative submission is normally seven months after enrolment. A portfolio with documentary evidence is a favoured APL assessment tool in the UK, (Hemsworth, 2007 and Pokorny, 2012). Candidates include evidence such as testimonials, certificates of attendance or achievement from work place events, sometimes an extended curriculum vitae as well as the reflective narrative. The educational adviser marks and grades the work. It is then moderated and the process overseen by an external examiner. The result is read at an examination board and the APL candidate receives notification of achievement with a transcript. These processes are consistent with the QAA (2004) Guidelines on the Accreditation of Prior Learning and the emerging updated UK Quality Code for Higher Education (2011).

APL AND PRE-REGISTRATION NURSING

Students undertaking a pre-registration nursing programme in the UK today will be prepared to either the NMC 2004 or 2010 professional standards for competence and education. Some students will be registering with the NMC with a diploma level qualification if they were taught on a curriculum that pre-dated the new standards published in September 2010. By September 2013 all courses will lead to a graduate registration only (NMC, 2010b). Under the statute the Nursing and Midwifery Order 2001 standards are required to set a minimal level for programme providers, normally HEIs, to determine programme content, learning outcomes and assessment criteria. The standards are underpinned by requirements and all must be fully demonstrated to meet the standards, (NMC, 2010a).

KEY LEARNING ACTIVITY 9

For context, look at the NMC 2004 *Standards of proficiency for pre-registration nursing education* and in particular standards 3, 4 and 5. These can be obtained from the NMC website http://www.nmc-uk.org/Educators/ in the 'Educators' section:

- Note the minimum length of the pre-registration course if previous academic and experiential learning is recognized.
- Note the appropriate prior learning and experience that can be considered and the definition for advanced standing.
- What has to be mapped for quality assurance purposes?

There are several things to highlight from this learning activity. Firstly, the one third rule and applicants have typically presented with an array of qualifications in the past as acknowledged by Scott (2010). Not all are credit bearing and so some HEIs, including the author's own, work with a tariff system. In effect, the admissions tutor, APL co-ordinator and course leader have predetermined the equivalence of the prior learning in terms of volume of credit, academic level and its match to learning outcomes and standards of proficiency. The tariff is driven by both national trends and local provision; courses studied at Further Education (FE) colleges including Foundation Degrees and apprenticeship type schemes run by NHS or health care employers. This mechanism is well suited to the structure of the MAD and NMC 2004 curricula which have a defined common foundation programme at the start of the programme at certificate level 4, (QAA, 2008). Secondly, the NMC as the regulator stipulate that evidence must be available to show how the APL meets the common foundation programme outcomes and the standards beyond the first year. Thirdly, the mapping process as an APL mechanism must be approved by the NMC as part of course approval. For further explanation of Foundation Degrees see the QAA benchmarks updated in 2010. These degrees were introduced in 2000 and contribute to widening participation.

New guidance

As previously mentioned new standards for pre-registration nursing education were published in 2010. Early in 2011 the NMC issued guidance on APL for existing courses which came into line with the new curriculum (NMC, circular 01/2011 and NMC, 2010a). There are some notable changes which create tensions for higher education including the bestowing of academic awards. HEIs have rules about how much APL can contribute to a named degree such as Bachelor of Science (BSc) with honours (Johnson, 2002 and Hemsworth, 2007). There is often no APL in the final year when credit is achieved at level 6 and includes a substantive piece of work such as a dissertation. See Chapter 1 for a reminder of the academic levels.

Before the next learning activity it is important to highlight some other changes with the new standards. There is no common foundation programme and nursing students have to meet competencies which are general and *field* specific. The competencies replace what were known as 'proficiencies' and are grouped into four domains:

- professional values
- communication and interpersonal skills
- nursing practice and decision-making
- leadership, management and team working.

The NMC use the following definition of competence:

the combination of skills, knowledge and attitudes, values and technical abilities that underpin safe and effective nursing practice and interventions (adapted from Queensland Nursing Council 2009).

NMC (2010a:11)

The four fields replace the 'branches' and are described by the NMC in Figure 3.1 (NMC, 2010b):

FIGURE 3.1 The four fields of nursing

Adult nurses focus mainly on caring for people who are 18 or over who are ill, recovering from an accident or illness, or learning to live with a disability. They also keep people mentally and physically healthy.

Mental health nurses provide care to people of all ages, including children, who experience or may be at risk of developing mental health problems. Like nurses in other fields, they provide nursing care and treatment to support people's physical, psychological, social, mental and spiritual health and recovery.

Learning disabilities nurses care for people of all ages, including children, with a learning disability, aiming to ensure they can maximize their health and independence. This includes working closely with people with learning disabilities their families and carers and providing care and advice in meeting challenging and complex needs.

Children's nurses care for children and young people, from birth to mid to late teens, in a wide range of healthcare and community settings. They work in partnership with children and young people, and their families, to plan their care, negotiate who will give that care and when and where is should be provided. They work to promote healthy behaviours and prevent ill health and seek to protect them from abuse and neglect.

From: Nursing & Midwifery Council. 2010b. *Pre-registration nursing education in the UK*. Page 5.

KEY LEARNING ACTIVITY 10

Look at the NMC 2010a *Standards for Pre-registration Nursing Education*. These can be obtained from the NMC website http://www.nmc-uk.org/Educators/ in the 'Educators' section. There are ten standards for education for programme approval and delivery. Find standard three for *selection, admission, progression and completion*:

- Expand the 'requirements' section at 3.5: *Programme providers must ensure that programmes include opportunities for accreditation of prior learning (APL)*. The NMC uses the term Approved Education Institution (AEI) instead of HEI.
- Note the six requirements. The first (3.5.1) has further 'guidance' statements.
- Check how much APL is allowed within a programme. See requirement 3.5.2.
- What if you are a midwife or already have a registration as a nurse with the NMC? See requirements 3.5.5 and 3.5.6.

The standard indicates that APL up to a maximum of 50 per cent is allowed (requirement 3.5.2) providing all the programme requirements can be met. This includes an applicant who is a NMC registered midwife (requirement 3.5.6).

Requirement 3.5.3 reminds programme providers of the need to comply with Article 31 of Directive 2005/36/EC which is about recognition of professional qualifications across the European Community. This stipulates the number of hours for theory and practice (4600) and the content of programmes for 'general care' and so affects the adult field applicants.

Nurses who are already on the register and want to qualify in a different field of practice can be considered for *unlimited* APL (requirement 3.5.5) providing programme requirements are met. The latter presents challenges for several reasons although the NMC does acknowledge that 100 per cent APL is unlikely:

1 An applicant already on the NMC register is not usually eligible for a second student grant from public money for the duration of the programme. HEIs may not allow a student to self finance when places on the course are commissioned by the NHS. The emerging plans for workforce design will influence developments around commissions and early indications point to fewer places (DH, 2012).

2 If an applicant is not eligible for a grant in a different field of practice employer secondment is an option. It is very costly for the employer to pay a salary and pay the course fees if the member of staff is then placed elsewhere to obtain relevant experience and practice hours.

3 If the applicant already has a degree leading to registration in one field of nursing practice what academic award should be awarded for the second field of practice? The NMC have stipulated this should be at degree level but unlimited APL runs the risk of 'double-counting' credit. Programme providers need to ensure there is an exit award such as a Graduate Certificate (60 credits at level 6) or a postgraduate award for nursing graduates qualifying in a second field of practice. For consistency this should be incorporated within the programme design as the NMC stipulate the approach should *be to develop a single programme with different pathways* (NMC, 2010c: 31)

How to use APL

The NMC does provide advice and support as to how APL should be applied within pre-registration nursing education (NMC, 2010c). Standard three is clear about having rigorous processes for accrediting prior learning and experience (requirement 3.5.1). The emphasis is on using systems that are compliant with the best practice guidelines (QAA, 2004). The guidance statement G3.5.1a (NMC, 2010a) gives four indications for when APL should be applied for accrediting previous learning:

● starting a programme

● transferring from one AEI to another

● moving from one nursing field to another

● returning to a programme after a lengthy break.

The advice is to embed APL within selection and admission processes and take an individual or collective approach. The collective approach could include the use of a tariff system mentioned earlier. Particular courses such as a relevant Foundation Degree can be mapped to the programme requirements in terms of practice and theory hours and the general and field specific competencies across the four domains. (Subject specific benchmark statements might be equally relevant.) Overseas qualifications also have to be checked for equivalence. Some AEIs use their collective expertise accrued through student admissions and registration services. Others will refer to the National Recognition Information Centre for the United Kingdom database (NARIC – http://www.naric.org.uk/). The individual approach can be more resource intensive, one of the criticisms of APL and its processes. Applicants do, however, have unique experiences and that might include an interrupted programme of study due to illness or pregnancy. Applicants can return after a lengthy break providing the qualification is achieved within five years as a full-time student or seven years as a part-time student, (NMC, 2010c). This reinforces the currency of the learning and achievement.

It is worth noting that applicants transferring, moving from one nursing field or returning, are likely to have prior learning with credit and experience generated from a diploma style curriculum. So it is important that this is mapped to the new fields of nursing practice with their generic and field specific competencies to be valid. Whereas AEIs cannot entertain bespoke courses for large numbers of applicants with APL there are mechanisms for ensuring transparent and robust processes. Figures 3.2 and 3.3 demonstrate an individual approach and are used as guidance for applicants in one AEI. The established mechanisms for experiential learning used by qualified nurses can equally be applied to pre-registration nursing applicants. The flow chart in Figure 3.2 refers to CRB checks. This is the Criminal Records Bureau which is an executive agency of the Home Office to ensure safer recruitment and protection of patients and clients.

FIGURE 3.2 Guidance for applicants seeking APL

From the School of Nursing & Midwifery, University of Brighton web pages

All claims for APL will be considered on an individual basis by the admissions tutor in conjunction with the course leader and APL Co-ordinator.

1   Applicants must make a make a UCAS application and be interviewed in the normal manner. The prior learning should be indicated on the application form **within the personal statement**.

2   Prior learning and experience will be discussed at interview. Original transcripts and course certificates must be seen including evidence of NMC registration if applicable. Overseas qualifications will be checked for equivalence. Transcripts in English with verified translation may be required.

3   The outcome of selection will be notified together with a decision about what point the successful applicant would join the pre-registration nursing course, for example, beginning of year two of the programme.

4   Where an applicant is offered a place on the course subject to evidence of learning from experience, the individual may be asked to provide a portfolio of evidence for this APL claim. This would be a conditional offer. Evidence must be mapped against the requirements of the pre-registration nursing course.

5   A half day workshop is available to assist with the mapping process. **There is a charge for this workshop** which includes the guidance of an educational adviser for submission of the APL claim to an examination board. **There is a further charge for submission and marking of the APL claim.** Information about costs and booking places on the workshop can be found on the Study Days and Workshop web page at: http://www.brighton.ac.uk/hss/study-days/

6   Once the APL claim has been achieved, the applicant will be informed at what point they would join the pre-registration nursing course, for example, beginning of year three of the programme. Please see flow chart.

It also mentions second level nurses which refers to enrolled nurses who have undertaken a shorter two year programme leading to professional registration. State enrolled nurses first appeared in 1943 when they were originally known as assistant nurses. By the early 1990s programmes had ceased as the recommendation was for one level of entry to the profession (UKCC, 1986).

The flow chart in Figure 3.3 mentions 'progression point' within the successful outcome box. The new curriculum has two progression points which divide the programme into three parts. Each progression point has a set of criteria which are matched to the four competency domains, (NMC, 2010a: Annexe 2 pages 97–102). These can be used within a standardized template for APL applicants to demonstrate where previous learning and experience matches. This fulfils requirement 3.5.4 in relation to mapping students who transfer between AEIs. It can also be used for the other APL indications and incorporate the five *Essential Skills Clusters (ESC)*. The ESC were originally introduced in 2008 and support the achievement of competencies (NMC, 2010a: Annexe 3 pages 103–143) and are:

- care, compassion and communication
- organizational aspects of care
- infection prevention and control
- nutrition and fluid management
- medicines management.

Of course, much of this is supposition as the new standards for pre-registration nursing education are newly implemented with the first AEIs having received programme approval to commence courses in 2011/12. This highlights the importance of calibrating your practice as an APL practitioner. The APL Network of the Southern England Consortium for Credit Accumulation and Transfer (**SEEC**) held a professional development seminar for the Nursing Profession in September 2011. It was attended by nurse educators from England, Scotland and Wales who are admissions tutors, field leaders, APL co-ordinators and course leaders. An adviser from the NMC also attended to talk about the new standards but the most useful discussion centred on case study examples so that educators could share practice and learn from one another. There will be a follow up seminar in 2013 to see what colleagues have learned from experience.

FIGURE 3.3 **FLOW CHART** for Accreditation of Prior Learning (APL) in Pre-Registration Nursing

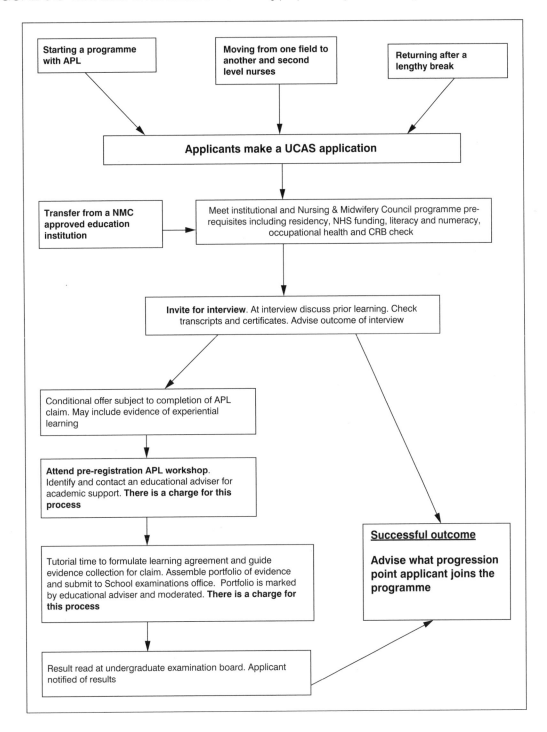

SUMMARY

The aim of this chapter was to explore how APL has been used within nursing. By looking at the changes to nurse education and its subsequent move to the higher education sector, it is easy to see how APL has been used by nurses to 'catch up' with academic achievement. At the same time it has allowed access to higher education that might not have been available through traditional routes to undergraduate studies. The lessons learned and the expertise gained is now being applied to changes within pre-registration nursing education.

Widening participation and recognition of prior learning are embraced to a much greater extent. With that come challenges to meet the requirements of higher education institutions and the professional, statutory and regulatory body (PSRB) the Nursing & Midwifery Council. This Chapter has engaged with some of the debates around APL and its application to pre-registration nursing education. It has offered some solutions but tensions remain at a time when more change is expected from NHS, higher education and PSRB reform.

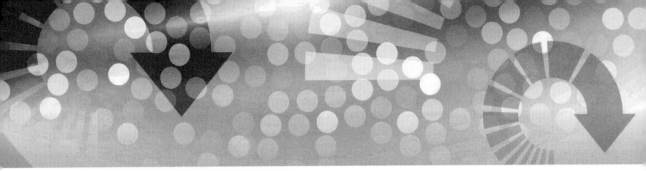

CHAPTER 4
PRIOR LEARNING ASSESSMENT AND RECOGNITION (PLAR): A CASE STUDY OF A HUMAN SERVICE PROGRAMME IN CANADA

INTRODUCTION

Prior Learning Assessment and Recognition has been taking place in Canada since the 1970s. This chapter will examine the practice of prior learning assessment within a human service programme at a community college in the province of Ontario, Canada. The approach taken is 'bottom-up' analysis, as referred to in Chapter 1, and the focus is squarely on the practice of prior learning assessment and recognition, henceforth referred to as PLAR – the term and acronym currently in use in Canada.[1]

---

[1]Prior Learning Assessment and Recognition (PLAR) is the current term/acronym used in Canada but it is gradually undergoing a change to Recognition of Prior Learning (RPL).

The practice of recognizing prior learning at a Canadian college will be explored using a case study. Firstly, the underlying definitions, assumptions, and principles of PLAR within the Canadian context will be stated. Next, an overview of the process that adults (henceforth referred to as PLAR candidates) go through when seeking recognition for their prior learning at a community college will be presented. Then, an in-depth case study will be used to examine PLAR practice using a developmental or holistic approach. The roles of the PLAR advisor and assessor (PLAR practitioner) and the PLAR candidate will be discussed. The case study is about the journey of a gentleman named Neil who utilized the PLAR and portfolio development process to successfully navigate through a transition period in his life and chart a new course for him and his family. Included in reviewing Neil's path will be a look at the steps, the challenges, and the benefits he experienced.

At the end of this Chapter, the reader will be able to:

- Define PLAR, its assumptions, methods and principles.

- Describe the holistic approach as it pertains to the use of PLAR in a social services programme.

- Identify the stages of PLAR and portfolio development.

- Describe the roles of the PLAR Advisor and Assessor.

- State the challenges and benefits of undertaking a PLAR process.

THE FOUNDATION OF PLAR PRACTICE IN THE SOCIAL SERVICE WORKER PROGRAMME

The practice of prior learning assessment in the Social Service Worker programme (SSW) at Loyalist College in Belleville, Canada is based on the principles of adult learning and commonly accepted definitions, assumptions and principles of PLAR in Canada. These principles and the practice of prior learning assessment were introduced to the programme by Paul Zakos, the first coordinator and one of the developers of the SSW programme. His work at First Nations Technical Institute (1985–2012) and that of his colleagues at FNTI had a major influence on the development of the holistic approach to PLAR at Loyalist College and across Canada. The principles of adult learning, which underlie and are deeply embedded in the delivery of the SSW programme, are based on the theory of adult learning (andragogy) developed by Malcolm Knowles (1980) as well as the work of Carl Rogers (1969), as referred to in Chapter 1. The often-cited definition of PLAR is:

a systematic process that involves the identification, documentation, assessment and recognition of learning. This learning may be acquired through formal and informal study including work and life experience, training, independent study, volunteer work, travel, hobbies and family experiences.

Day (2000)

PLAR is also based on a set of assumptions. These are:

1   Adults do acquire college level learning outside the classroom.
2   This learning should be assessed for credit where appropriate.
3   To require adults to repeat courses in which they have previously acquired the learning is disrespectful, costly and inefficient.
4   PLAR should be accessible to all qualified individuals.

5 PLAR services should be visible and well advertized.

6 The assessment of prior learning should be conducted using the same standards and outcomes as in-class learners.

PLAR is based on a set of underlying principles identified by Whitaker, 1989. These include, but are not limited to the following:

1 Credit should be awarded for *learning not experience*.

2 Learning must be proven using an appropriate method of assessment.

3 Learning must be at a college level.

4 Learning must contain a mix of theory and practice appropriate to the subject.

5 Learning must be assessed and credit awarded by a subject matter expert (faculty).

A key point is that *what is learned*, that is, what a learner knows and can do, is more important than where or how it was learned. In addition the assessment process that must be deemed to be valid, reliable, authentic and rigorous (Chapter 1, pp. 6–7).

The methods of prior learning assessment can include portfolio review, skills demonstrations, challenge exams, oral exams, project and product assessments, standardized tests and programme review. For the purposes of this case study, a portfolio-assisted PLAR process will be used and examined.

PLAR practice is also based upon the established guidelines created by the US based Council for Adult and Experiential Learning (CAEL) (Whitaker, 1989). The Ten Standards for Assessing Learning for Credit have long been the guide to prior learning assessment work world-wide. In Canada, a set of minimum standards for PLAR were developed in 1997 by the Canadian Labour Force Development Board (CLFDB). (Chapter 1, p. 9) Both the CAEL and CLFDB standards of practice form the foundation for the standards of practice for PLAR in the SSW programme at Loyalist College and in many institutions across Canada.

There are two broad approaches to PLAR: the technical approach and the holistic approach. The technical approach is primarily content based and the assessment tends to be summative. Generally little to no personal reflection or reflective writing is required. Technical assessment involves providing evidence/ documentation specifically related to the competencies or learning outcomes of a course. It is evidence or fact based and structured. Personal and life experiences are less significant, reflection is minimal, and education and career planning tends not to be a part of the assessment process.

The holistic approach is broader, more flexible and more comprehensive. Learning is viewed as lifelong and life-wide. The assessment process is both formative and summative in nature. This approach is fully learner or candidate-centered. It takes into account the candidate's experiences, needs and goals. It actively engages the candidate in all aspects of the portfolio development and assessment process. It is also a collaborative process whereby the candidate works through the PLAR process with an advisor and programme faculty as needed. This approach requires the candidate to produce evidence/documentation of competencies achieved by way of a portfolio.

THE HOLISTIC APPROACH

The approach to assessing prior learning in the SSW programme is a holistic approach. It is comprehensive in nature and involves both the recognition of prior experiential learning as well as transfer of courses/credits from other post-secondary institutions. The approach is both a process and a product. It recognizes that significant learning is acquired through life and work experiences as well as formal education. The process aspect of the holistic approach involves the development of a relationship between the PLAR practitioner (advisor/assessor) and the PLAR candidate (adult learner). The relationship develops over a period of time whereby the PLAR practitioner first takes on the role of advisor and guides and assists the candidate in compiling a portfolio and encourages the candidate to reflect upon his/her life and work experiences and to document those experiences. This is a formative assessment process, both for the advisor and the learner. It leads to rich learning and insight on the part of the learner and often times for the advisor! The process eventually leads to the product – the completion of a portfolio which is submitted for assessment. At this point, the advisor becomes the assessor and summatively assesses the portfolio for credits and assigns a final grade for each course challenged. In this case study, the advisor becomes the assessor once the completed portfolio is submitted, but it is not always the case that one person fulfils both roles. Sometimes the advisor and assessor are two different people.

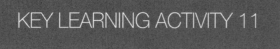

KEY LEARNING ACTIVITY 11

Holistic Versus Technical Approach

Identify the key difference between the holistic approach to PLAR/RPL and the technical approach to PLAR/RPL.

> What challenges or tension do you foresee in implementing a holistic approach in your programme or institution?

> State one strategy you could attempt that might ease or help overcome challenges towards a holistic PLAR/RPL approach?

OVERVIEW OF THE PLAR PROCESS

An overview of the PLAR process as practiced in the SSW programme at Loyalist College is shown in Figure 4.1.

The PLAR process begins with a preliminary step whereby the advisor provides information about the process, roles, costs, the development of a portfolio, how it will be assessed and further course planning. Upon receiving information about how the process works, the candidate has the opportunity to ask the advisor questions and to seek clarification or elaboration as to what is involved. He/she then decides whether or not to proceed. After deciding to go through the process, the candidate then meets with the advisor and begins a conversation about the programme and the courses within that programme to determine which courses he/she might seek recognition for. The advisor and the candidate begin to discuss what a portfolio is and how to compile one. They discuss different types of documentation and how to organize it in relation to specific courses being challenged by the candidate. The advisor and candidate meet to discuss the portfolio as it is being developed. The advisor assists the candidate with assembling his/her portfolio in the recommended format. These meetings help the candidate stay on track and to build momentum and confidence in the process. Eventually, the candidate completes his/her portfolio and submits it for review, assessment, and determination of credits to the programme faculty who are subject-matter experts. The faculty has the authority to award credits for prior learning as well as to assign a grade for each credit earned. At Loyalist College, the dean of the School of Human Studies approves all prior learning assessments. Generally, faculty assessors review the portfolio and have a subsequent meeting with the candidate to discuss the portfolio and outcome of the review. At this time, a plan is developed to complete the remaining required courses in the programme.

Alternatively, candidates are advised to take a Portfolio Development course, a credit course, to receive assistance in developing a portfolio for the PLAR process. The course is 28 hours and is offered online over a three month period.

CONTEXT FOR THE CASE STUDY

The setting for this case study is in a small community college – Loyalist College of Applied Arts and Technology – located in Belleville (population 45 000), in the province of Ontario, Canada. Loyalist College

FIGURE 4.1 PLAR Process in the SSW

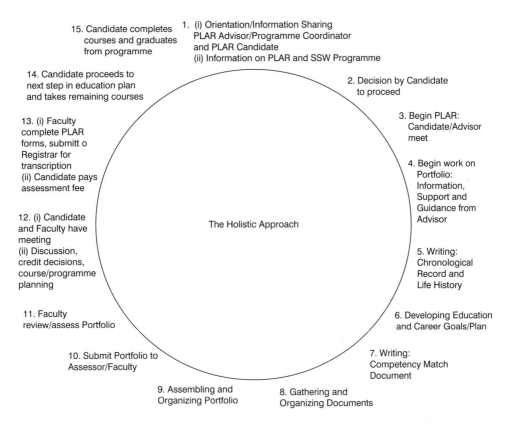

15. Candidate completes courses and graduates from programme

1. (i) Orientation/Information Sharing PLAR Advisor/Programme Coordinator and PLAR Candidate (ii) Information on PLAR and SSW Programme

14. Candidate proceeds to next step in education plan and takes remaining courses

2. Decision by Candidate to proceed

13. (i) Faculty complete PLAR forms, submitt o Registrar for transcription (ii) Candidate pays assessment fee

3. Begin PLAR: Candidate/Advisor meet

4. Begin work on Portfolio: Information, Support and Guidance from Advisor

12. (i) Candidate and Faculty have meeting (ii) Discussion, credit decisions, course/programme planning

The Holistic Approach

5. Writing: Chronological Record and Life History

11. Faculty review/assess Portfolio

6. Developing Education and Career Goals/Plan

10. Submit Portfolio to Assessor/Faculty

7. Writing: Competency Match Document

9. Assembling and Organizing Portfolio

8. Gathering and Organizing Documents

has a student body of 3000 full-time students and is the fifth smallest college out of 25 colleges in Ontario. In total there are 62 post-secondary diploma programme at the college. Loyalist College has an approved PLAR policy (2009) which recognizes and supports PLAR activity, and states that individuals can seek recognition (credit) for their prior learning from a qualified faculty in any programme. The policy further states that individuals can seek credit up to 75 per cent of courses within a programme. A minimum of 25 per cent of the course load must be taken at the college in order to receive a diploma from the college. Loyalist College has well-established administration procedures that support and accompany the PLAR process, such as information brochures, registration procedures and forms, recording of grades, transcripts and invoicing and collection of fees. Since 1979, Loyalist College has been assisting adult learners gain formal recognition for their prior learning. A significant amount of this activity has occurred in the Social Service Worker programme, and as a result there is a long-established process and several faculty trained in PLAR. The SSW programme is a two-year full-time programme which can also be taken on a part-time basis. There are a total of 24 courses within the programme and it is responsible for meeting provincial SSW vocational standards (Ministry of Training, Colleges and Universities, 2006). The profession of Social Service Worker is provincially regulated by the Ontario College of Social Workers and Social Service Workers (OCSWSSW).

The SSW programme uses a portfolio-assisted prior learning assessment process. This includes the development and submission of a portfolio for review as well as an interview with faculty to determine the outcome of the request for prior learning recognition. At the conclusion of the interview a plan is created with the candidate to facilitate the completion of the remaining courses for the diploma.

THE PLAR CANDIDATE

Thus far the theoretical and philosophical underpinnings of PLAR have been presented. But PLAR is not just about theories, processes, and policies. It is about *real people*. Adults who engage in a PLAR process are people who often share some common traits: they have considerable life and work experience and have rich experiential learning which equates to college or university level (or trades certification), they have families to support, they want to have some recognition for what they already know, they want to acquire a formal credential and not have to repeat things they already know (waste time), they want to move back into the workforce quickly (if they are unemployed) and they are highly goal oriented, focused and motivated, although they may be slightly fearful to return to formal education. In fact, these learners are additive to programmes they enroll in and are highly likely to complete the programmes they begin.

The person involved in this case study is Neil. (Neil is a real person and has given his consent to use his story and PLAR journey for this chapter and book). At the time of his PLAR experience he was in his early 30s, married, father of six young children and had been employed for nine years at a residential facility for youth. His previous education at the college-level was in an area unrelated to his work. His position at the youth facility (which he had obtained unexpectedly) had increasing responsibilities over time and he eventually became a supervisor of several group homes and staff. However, the agency was undergoing significant review and changes, and in time, Neil viewed his position as a 'dead end'. To him it was no longer challenging and there was little opportunity for advancement. His employment involved a great deal of shift work which was difficult on family life, particularly a young and large family. Without having a college Social Service Worker diploma (credential), Neil's opportunities both at the youth facility and in the field generally, were severely restricted. As a result, he began to research ways in which he could obtain a college diploma in social service work as expeditiously as possible.

NEIL'S PLAR JOURNEY

First meeting: sharing PLAR and programme information

Neil visited Loyalist College to see what programmes he would be best suited to enroll in. He met with the programme coordinator of the SSW programme and shared why he was there and what his life and work circumstances were. Neil indicated that he wanted to learn more about the programme and courses, what study options he had, where the diploma would lead him, how long it would take him to complete it, how much PLAR assessment and tuition costs, and finally how to go about receiving credit for his prior learning. The SSW coordinator was also a PLAR advisor/assessor and Neil eagerly listened to the programme information, how the PLAR process worked, and what he needed to do to fully participate in it. Neil was told that the process was both reflective and that it involved three components: Looking Back, Taking Stock and Looking Ahead. The Looking Back part involved reflecting on his life and work experiences as they related to the field of social service work. The Taking Stock part involved thinking about where his life was at now – what was good about it and what he would like to change. Finally, the Looking Ahead part was about setting new goals for his continued education and his career, and developing a plan to achieve them. The development of a portfolio was discussed along with how to compile one with the guidance and support of an advisor. Neil learned that a portfolio is a file, folder or binder that contains your prior learning achievements and education/vocation goals. It also specifies which courses you are seeking credit for and documentation to prove you have acquired the learning. Toward the end of the meeting, Neil enthusiastically agreed to become involved in the PLAR process and begin to develop his portfolio. His initial reaction was 'this doesn't seem like a lot of work, I'll have the portfolio completed and ready for assessment in no time'. A follow-up meeting with his PLAR advisor was arranged shortly thereafter.

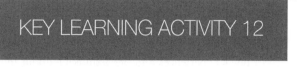

KEY LEARNING ACTIVITY 12

The Initial Interview

Getting to know the PLAR candidate is a fundamental aspect of the work. In the first meeting, building rapport and asking questions are very important.

Create 3–5 questions that will enable you to learn more about the candidate's prior work experience, current life circumstances and future education/career goals.

Second meeting: getting started

In between meetings, Neil, a self-described 'pack-rat', began to sort through a great deal of documentation at home which he had accumulated over many years. He began to select what he thought were the most relevant pieces to bring to the next meeting with his advisor. He managed to scale down his documents to two banker boxes, one hockey bag and a milk crate! Before discussing all of his documentation, Neil and his advisor first had an in-depth discussion about the SSW programme, the courses in the programme, and an overview of what was expected from those courses. Neil was also given a handout which described the competencies for each of the courses. This sharing of course information allowed Neil to begin to think about courses for which he had prior learning and could possibly challenge, as well as courses for which he had little or no prior knowledge, and should take. He was also made aware of the components of a portfolio, which included:

1   A chronological record
2   A life-history paper
3   A goals paper and education/career plan
4   An up-to-date resume
5   A competency match document
6   Support documentation.

Guidance and resource material would be provided for completion of each component. To assist in the compilation of the portfolio Neil was given a portfolio manual entitled *A Guide To Assist In The Preparation Of A Portfolio For Education, Vocational and Career Planning* (Zakos, FNTI, 2003).

During the meeting, Neil shared more about his field-related experiences including his various roles and duties within the agency, the extensive in-service training he had undertaken, as well as training he had delivered to staff. He also spoke about his other life experiences involving his family, volunteer work and church and community involvements. This led to a discussion about which documentation he could include in his portfolio. Neil indicated that he had a great deal and many types of documentation. Deciding on which pieces to use would be something to further consider.

Neil's reaction now was that the process seemed quite daunting but he was excited and willing to take on the challenge. The first step (and homework assignment) was to work on a Chronological Record.

The Chronological Record (CR) is a recollection and recording of significant life experiences. Some candidates choose to reflect back to their high school days while others choose to look further back than that. Neil was asked to list chronologically (year by year) important events or happenings in his life. The length of the paper is approximately one to two pages and it can be done in point form or chart form. The candidate has control over what to include in the CR and what to leave out. Generally, events or experiences included are:

1   Employment
2   Schools attended

3   Graduation
4   Seminars, workshops, conferences
5   Volunteer work
6   Travel
7   Major life events such as marriage, divorce, births, deaths, moving, etc.

The benefit of doing a CR is that it organizes all of one's experiences and one's thinking about them. It also provides the advisor with an overview of the candidate's experiences. It is a useful place to begin the PLAR process (Zakos, FNTI, 2003).

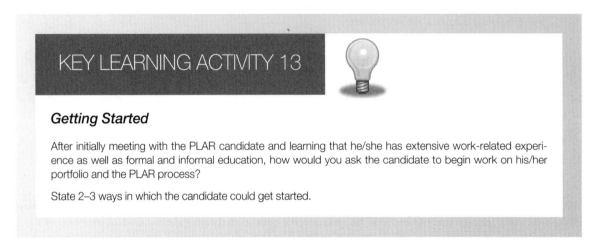

KEY LEARNING ACTIVITY 13

Getting Started

After initially meeting with the PLAR candidate and learning that he/she has extensive work-related experience as well as formal and informal education, how would you ask the candidate to begin work on his/her portfolio and the PLAR process?

State 2–3 ways in which the candidate could get started.

Third meeting: reflecting back and going deeper

Upon completing his CR and sharing it with his advisor, Neil was then asked to work on a Life History paper. The CR begins the process of Portfolio Thinking and allows for recollection of experiences and listing them chronologically but it doesn't account for what impact those experiences had on oneself, or what valuable learning could be derived from them. The process of writing a Life History paper – the next task – helps one gain a deeper awareness and understanding of oneself and how one has grown and changed (Zakos, FNTI, 2003). It enables the candidate 'to review the goals, decisions and learning that one has experienced and to review the ongoing development as a person' (Zakos, 2003). Often adults undervalue their life experiences and do not take the time out of their busy lives to reflect upon them. A Life History paper can reveal rich and often hidden learning, which occurs throughout one's life time.

Neil committed to working on his Life History paper as his next task in the PLAR process.

Fourth meeting: extracting learning from experience

Neil shared his completed Life History paper with his advisor and they discussed the significant life experiences, the learning he derived from them, how they related to social service work, and what documentation he could produce to support the learning.

One of the more difficult aspects of preparing a portfolio is determining how to organize each course challenge and deciding how much documentation is required as evidence to prove one's learning in a particular course. This component of the portfolio is known as the Competency Match Document (see Figure 4.2 – Zakos 2003). Neil was advised to complete the template by identifying experiences that relate to a specific course, and then glean learning from them. These experiences and learning require documentation as proof. Three diverse pieces of documentation would normally suffice for each course for which he was seeking a credit (the concept of **triangulation**) (Day, 2002). In addition to three pieces of documentation, Neil was asked to write a narrative outlining the context and extent of his related experiences as they pertained to the courses he was challenging.

FIGURE 4.2 Template for the Competency Match Document

Course Title: Course Competencies (or Learning Outcomes)

1 Narrative (describe the context and extent of experience related to this course)

2

Experience	Learning from Experience	Supporting Documentation

KEY LEARNING ACTIVITY 14

Documentation

The PLAR candidate has asked to discuss documentation: how much he/she should include and what types of documentation are acceptable or strong.

Identify the two main types of documentation and define the concept of triangulation. Create a list of documentation that could be considered either as acceptable evidence or strong evidence.

To ensure that Neil was on the right track with preparing his course challenges (he was doing multiple challenges) in his portfolio, he submitted a draft of one challenge to his advisor for feedback. The advisor reviewed his work and provided input on how to improve the narrative and whether his documentation was sufficient and directly related to the outcomes of the course. The advisor provided encouragement and support to continue with the course challenges and the development of his portfolio.

Once the Competency Match Document was completed, Neil was asked to reflect on and record his education and career goals. Goal setting is an essential aspect of the PLAR process as it encourages the candidate to create a roadmap for their future and build on what they have already achieved. Neil was encouraged to set his goals, both short-term (less than two years) and long term (two to five years) using the SMART principles – Specific, Measurable, Achievable, Realistic and Time-lined.

Final meeting: the assessment process and summative evaluation

When Neil completed all of the components of the portfolio and had properly organized it, it was ready to be submitted to programme faculty for assessment. In the SSW programme, two or three faculty members review the portfolio prior to the interview with the candidate, but do not share their observations with each other. When assessing the portfolio, the faculty considers the following principles/questions.

- Validity: Does the documentation relate to the competencies/learning outcomes for which credit is being sought? Does it match all or part of those competencies/learning outcomes for the course?

- Sufficiency: Can the documentation serve as conclusive proof for one or more of the courses being assessed? What else might be required?
- Currency: Is the documentation relatively recent and up-to-date in relation to the standards for the occupation/ programme?
- Authenticity: Is the direct evidence the work of the candidate? Does the evidence give an accurate picture to support his/her claims of competence?

The faculty panel met with Neil and a discussion ensued about the portfolio/PLAR process, the specific course challenges, the candidate's goals and finally about a plan to complete the remaining courses.

This meeting took about an hour and it was interactive. It was a summative evaluation of Neil's quest for prior learning recognition and credits. The interview was conducted in an open, friendly and respectful manner. The panel asked Neil further questions, sought clarification and elaboration. Neil also asked the panelists questions regarding the SSW programme and courses, the assessment process and about the portfolio development process.

In such meetings, decisions are made by the faculty panel, with the candidate present, about credit awards. However, grades for individual courses are assigned afterwards when the candidate has left the meeting so that the panelists can discuss the portfolio and their assessment decisions before reaching a consensus on the grades achieved. The standard used to evaluate learning is the same one applied to regular learners. If a passing grade is 60 per cent for an in-class learner, then the same applies to a PLAR candidate. If the panelists believe that some 'essential' learning is missing even though 60 per cent of the course outcomes have been achieved, the candidate will be advised to complete a learning contract to fill the gap. A learning contract is a formal, written agreement between the candidate and faculty to address a specific learning goal(s). Figure 4.3 is an example of a learning contract.

Towards the conclusion of the assessment interview, a plan is discussed and developed with the candidate about what courses are left to complete the diploma, when they are offered, and what is the most preferred way to complete them. In Neil's case, he successfully received credit for many of the courses in the SSW programme and a plan was put in place for Neil to complete the remaining courses.

After the interview, faculty completes the PLAR form which is sent to the dean of the School of Human Studies for approval. This form outlines the courses successfully challenged and credit awarded, the assigned

---

FIGURE 4.3 Learning Contract Template

Date: Learner:
Faculty:
Course:

Learning Outcomes	Resources/ Strategies	Assignments	Due Date	Evaluation

Final Grade:

The learning outcomes have been successfully achieved.

_____

Faculty

_____

Learner

grades, and which faculty conducted the assessment. The PLAR form, once signed by the dean, goes to the Registrar's Office to be recorded and fees correctly invoiced.

CHALLENGES OF PLAR

There are many challenges that can become a barrier to a PLAR service. Some of these include, though are not limited to: institutional or systemic issues, administrative or procedural barriers, policy shortcomings, faculty unwillingness or resistance to engage in PLAR, lack of PLAR training or insufficient resources and inflexible programmes. Loyalist College, over many years, has addressed (and continues to address) many of these barriers. PLAR candidates also experience challenges in undertaking a PLAR process. Just as each candidate is unique, so too are the challenges they face. Some of those challenges are:

1   Lack of time to work on a portfolio due to multiple responsibilities such as family, work, community, volunteer and other commitments.
2   Fear of failure and pressure to succeed.
3   Lack of confidence in returning to formal education.
4   Struggle with understanding 'edu-ease', education terminology and language used by staff in a college and/or in the college or programme print/web literature.
5   Fear of writing.
6   Unfamiliar with current technology.
7   Fear of getting started on portfolio.
8   Locating or gathering documentation.
9   Worried about not having enough or too much documentation.
10 Inability to extract or articulate learning from experiences.
11 Difficulty identifying or explaining the theory behind the practice/experience.
12 Feeling that life/work experiences are not worthy of recognition or college credit.
13 Deciding which courses to seek recognition/credit for and which ones to take.
14 Managing emotions when reflecting back on difficult or painful life experiences.

KEY LEARNING ACTIVITY 15

Barriers and Challenges

PLAR candidates face many barriers and challenges when engaging in a PLAR process. Some of these are intrapersonal and others are financial, environmental, or systemic.

Consider three or four barriers that have been presented. As their PLAR adviser, how would you assist them to overcome these barriers?

In Neil's case, he did experience challenges that had an influence on his PLAR journey. He indicated that some of his challenges were: initially having too much documentation, having to sort through and decide which were the most relevant pieces to include in his portfolio; at times he said he felt 'stuck' or at a roadblock before realizing that these were all junctures that lead to new stages of development and recognition; the process was emotionally draining at times especially when he reflected on difficult experiences or goals he hadn't achieved; it was challenging to find time to work on the portfolio because several concurrent life circumstances were impacting him (e.g., his wife was expecting a child soon to be born, his father was seriously ill, he had recently been laid off from work, and he was exploring education options).

The role of the PLAR advisor is particularly important during challenging times. They can keep the process moving forward in two ways: (1) by encouraging the candidate to persevere and stay the course and (2) by helping to alleviate or reduce the barriers which negatively impact the candidates. According to Morris Keeton it is essential that in order to have success in PLAR it is necessary to advocate for 'lowering the barriers and increasing the supports' for learners. It is critical to the advisor's role to be aware of the barriers, to discuss them with the candidate when they arise, and to work towards resolving them immediately.

BENEFITS OF PLAR

The benefits of PLAR, particularly when using a holistic approach, are far reaching. The benefits extend beyond the receipt of credits towards a college programme. They include the candidate and his family, the college and its programmes and faculty, the profession, and ultimately the community.

Neil identified several benefits of the PLAR process. They include:

1 Feeling valued and respected by programme faculty and the college. 'The PLAR process personally was very enriching and liberating'.
2 A process that was more 'intense and rewarding than predicted'.
3 Furthering education and completing a college diploma. It also inspired him to continue to work on a university degree.
4 Savings of time and money.
5 An acknowledgement that his life's experiences counted for something.
6 Increased self-knowledge and understanding. The process 'brought life experiences into focus and allowed a plan to manifest itself'. Neil realized that his current state wasn't a dead end but part of something bigger.
7 Resultant healing and closure to some unresolved personal experiences.
8 Helping to establish clear education and career goals and a plan to achieve them.
9 Feeling happier and more in control of his future as he pursued his education and career goals.
10 Increased employability.
11 Creating a portfolio which can be used for other purposes in the future (such as ongoing education and employment).
12 The experience was shared with spouse and his children who were highly supportive and interested in his journey. Neil stated that though the experience was at times 'trying', it also opened up opportunities for discussion within his family.
13 The process has 'ripple effects'. Neil stated that his family gained a new appreciation for the value of education and educational experiences through observing and participating in his PLAR experience.
14 The PLAR process inspired Neil to work on a Legacy Book with his dying father.

The SSW programme also benefitted from Neil's participation in the PLAR process. They acquired a highly motivated and focused learner. Furthermore, Neil's recent field-related experience contributed to valuable discussions between Neil and faculty as well as Neil and his classmates. And lastly, having experienced, competent and driven candidates forces faculty to clearly communicate the course content, the learning outcomes, and the methods used to assess learning.

SUMMARY

Neil's story, in many ways, is similar to hundreds of adult learners who have participated in the PLAR process in the SSW programme over the past 30 years. The PLAR process utilizes a holistic approach which leads to positive outcomes for most candidates. However, not all PLAR candidates want or need the holistic approach. For example, those seeking only one course credit have a less comprehensive process, and a more streamlined technical approach is available for them. Candidates that do participate in a comprehensive portfolio development process, state that it is time-consuming, highly reflective and rigorous, and overall found it to be beneficial and worthwhile.

A post-script to Neil's PLAR story is the positive effect it had on his life and goals in subsequent years. Since undertaking the prior learning assessment process four years ago, Neil went on to complete the SSW programme and diploma. He re-entered the social services field and accepted an invitation to teach part-time at the college. He re-developed and submitted his portfolio for academic credit at a university and began working towards a degree. Finally, in the summer of 2011, Neil applied for and received a full-time professor position at Loyalist College.

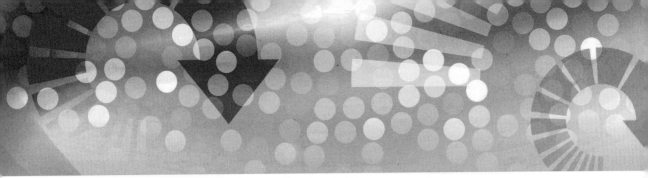

CHAPTER 5
ASSESSMENT OF
PRIOR LEARNING IN
THE US

The nature of modern American society has become more complex and interdependent; changes in competition, technology, information processing and lifestyles are all interacting to affect the way we lead our personal and professional lives. Continuous lifelong learning is essential for the development of strong economies necessary to compete in a global market place. New partnerships and alliances between educational institutions and host of organizations are blurring traditional educational boundaries. State policy makers are placing increased pressure on post-secondary institutions to increase the number of graduates if the US is to compete in global market place (Wertheim, 2009). These forces have converged to place increased pressure on colleges and universities to face the reality of change and embrace new processes and approaches to teaching and learning. The new paradigm often referred to as the learning paradigm, shifts the focus on learning acquired by the learner and away from the delivery of instruction by academic experts. What appears to be a subtle difference has immense impact on educational institutions. How students master competencies becomes the crucial emphasis, not where or who delivers the instruction. This shift requires a far more collaborative approach between educational institutions and learners. Placing more emphasis on learning and less importance of who delivers the learning has resulted in colleges and universities not being the only institutions involved in facilitating and supporting lifelong learning. The key features of continuous lifelong learning that colleges and universities need to address are open and flexible access, the growth of learning networks and partnerships and the recognition of learning wherever it takes place (the assessment of prior learning).

At the end of this Chapter, the reader will be able to:

● Define prior learning assessment in the United States.

● Explain the focus of prior learning assessment in the US.

● Trace the historical developments of prior learning assessment in the United States.

● Explain the educative rationale for assessing prior learning and its link to experiential learning.

● Define the primary methods and the impact on adult learners in the US.

● Identify the key components necessary to design a comprehensive prior learning assessment programme.

● Explain the importance of educational planning to the design and implementation of prior learning assessment.

This chapter will focus on the development of prior learning assessment in the United States. Prior learning assessment is a process of evaluating and granting college credit for learning that has taken place outside of academic control, using such methods as examination, programme evaluation and individualized approaches using a portfolio. The primary focus on the assessment of prior learning has opened access to higher education institutions for adult learners to both encourage and complete academic credentials.

HISTORICAL DEVELOPMENTS

The award of college credit for prior learning has grown from an experimental project to a recognized programme designed to assist adult learners in complete post-secondary academic degrees. The initial focus was on testing and programme evaluation growing out of the need to serve the increasing number of military personnel seeking college degrees. The first formal system for assessing prior learning in the United States was the General Educational Development Examination (GED). This programme was designed during World War II under the oversight of the American Council on Education (ACE) to assess the educational growth of service men and women who had left high school to serve in the armed forces. After the war, ACE extended the programme, using the GED examinations to demonstrate high-school equivalency for the civilian population. Before the end of World War II, the Educational Testing Service (ETS) of Princeton, New Jersey and ACE began evaluating military training and experience to determine civilian educational equivalency (American Council on Education, 2001). By 1947, ACE and the Department of Defense undertook a more ambitious project to evaluate the military occupational specialties (MOS) and training conducted by the armed forces to determine their comparability to college and university courses (American Council on Education, 2001). Using college and university faculty and staff, ACE established guidelines, procedures, and criteria for assessing both military training programmes and occupational specialties. Where equivalency to college courses existed, they recommended that colleges and universities consider awarding appropriate credit hours to the military personnel who had completed the trainings or attained the military occupational specialty levels. ACE established guidelines for colleges and universities to use in awarding the credit and worked with GIs to petition for that credit at various colleges and universities. Today, ACE's credit recommendation for military experiences is recognized at most colleges and universities.

A parallel project aimed at helping colleges and universities respond to adult students returning from the armed services was developed by the United States Armed Forces Institute (USAFI). During the war, USAFI provided correspondence courses and other educational materials to soldiers. Once the war was over USAFI also began offering testing and accreditation services to parlay learning soldiers had acquired into currency recognizable and creditable by high schools and colleges. The DSST examination programme was opened to civilian personnel in the early 1990s. Today they offer 38 standardized exams in college subject areas such as Social Sciences, Math, Applied Technology, Business, Physical Sciences and Humanities; the exams are recognized at over 2000 institutions (About DSST, 2012).

In the mid-60s the College-Level Examination Program (CLEP) developed a widely used examination programme. CLEP exams test mastery of college level material acquired in a variety of ways outside the sponsorship of educational institutions. Exams are taken by adults just entering or returning to school, military service members and traditional college students looking for ways to shorten the time to complete their academic degrees. The exams are accepted by 2900 colleges and universities (CLEP, 2012).

Several early experiments linking the assessment of prior learning with accelerated degree programmes for adults on the collegiate front were conducted. In 1954, Brooklyn College was perhaps the first to award credits directly to adults on the basis of the assessment of previous learning experiences using an individualized portfolio as the primary tool (Gamson, 1989). The University of Oklahoma in 1957 designed one of the first baccalaureate programmes for adults. In 1963, Queens College, City University of New York (CUNY) began a special programme for adults – the Adult Collegiate Education Program – which gave formal recognition, in the form of credit, to adult students for what they had learned through their life and work experiences. In the following years, Florida International University, Antioch College, Goddard College, and several other colleges developed unique programmes for adult students and mechanisms for recognizing and crediting their prior experiential learning. Assessment opportunities for adults began to become more prevalent in higher education during the late 1960s and early 1970s. The social, economic and educational pressures coupled with the decline in enrollments of the traditional age student contributed to not only the increase in adult students but the necessity of higher education to design programmes to attract and retain this growing group of non-traditional learners (Bamford-Rees, 2009). By the early 90s the number of part-time adult learners, enrolled in American colleges and universities had almost tripled, growing to almost 6 million (National University Continuing Education Association, 1990). In recent years, the percentage increase in the number of students age 25 and over has been larger than the percentage increase in the number of younger students, and this pattern is expected to continue (Fast Facts, 2011).

While a variety of non-traditional programmes had been established by the early 1970s, the pivotal influence on the development of prior leaning recognition programmes evolved from the Commission on Traditional Study. The Commission was a joint project of the Educational Testing Service (ETS) and the College Board. The commission recommended that colleges and universities make themselves more accessible to adult and part-time students by creating alternative avenues by which students could earn degrees (Gamson, 1989). More importantly, the commission emphasized the need to develop a variety of new ways to assess what students learned from life experiences. In 1974, based on the Commission's findings a small group of colleges and universities formed the Cooperative Assessment of Experiential Learning (CAEL) to develop and implement good practices regarding the awarding of college credit for non-academic learning experiences, placing particular emphasis on the development of the portfolio process. Early CAEL associates served the dual role of educators and change agents to both promote and develop methods to assess prior learning. This early work legitimized the assessment of prior learning by grounding the assessment practices in sound principles and established a systematic basis for standards, principles and practice. CAEL's standards of good practice have been adopted by regional accreditation bodies as well as colleges and universities both in the states and internationally. In 2006 the principles were revised to highlight the importance of learning how to learn well from experience and broadened the application of assessment from academic credentialing to other contexts; additional emphasis was placed on the need for ongoing attention to development of assessors (Fiddler and Marienau, 2009). CAEL (now called the Council for Adult and Experiential Learning) continues as an active non-profit organization working at all levels within the higher education, public, and private sectors to make it easier for people to get the education and training they need (CAEL What We Do, 2011).

DEFINITION, RATIONALE AND SCOPE OF PRIOR LEARNING ASSESSMENT

As stated, in the United States prior learning assessment is a process of evaluating and granting college credit for learning that has taken place outside of academic control using testing, programme evaluation and portfolios as the primary assessment tools. Prior learning is defined as the learning acquired from non-academic life or work experience that has occurred prior to formal contact with a college or university. Adults are often involved in a variety of learning activities that are not sponsored or directed by higher education. The types of learning activities are endless and the oversight of the activities is equally varied. A great deal of learning is occurring in the workplace – the American Society for Training and Development (ASTD) estimated that business and industry spends $125 billion annually on training and development (Stern, 2011). Adults participate in diverse, non-formal learning activities that they organize and conduct. Alan Tough's early study of adult learners found that 90 per cent of adults are involved in at least one learning activity annually, and the average learner conducts five learning activities, investing an average of 100 hours per learning effort and plans 80 per cent of the learning programme (Tough, 1971).

Three underlying arguments have contributed to the growth of assessment of prior learning programmes; the democratization of higher education, growth of experiential learning and the increasing need for an educated workforce. As the idea of a more democratic higher education system began to enter the public consciousness in the 1960s expanding educational opportunities for all, individuals and organizations began to question the status quo of how learners achieved an education (Gamson, 1989). We live in a society not only where credentials are increasingly important, but also where the alternatives for people without credentials is limited. Access to the credentialing process is largely contingent on the amount of higher education an individual has completed. Possession of a post-secondary degree enhances an individual's access to power and impacts almost every phase of life, affecting confidence, competence, advancement and income. Colleges and universities have expanded policies and created programmes and services with the goal of making the academy more accessible to a more diverse group of students. Prior learning assessment has been viewed as an important means of increasing access to higher education for people whom by virtue of their age, gender, race, socioeconomic background and/or prior educational qualifications have found it difficult to gain entry. More recently, the application of the assessment of prior learning has expanded as a means of gaining entry to professions, to jobs and employment progressions and to training and development opportunities by employees. It is increasingly linked with notions of economic regeneration and retraining, as well as the need for continuing education necessary to cope with the technological changes and the needs of the knowledge explosion (Wertheim, 2009).

The educative rationale for prior learning assessment is grounded in the experiential learning theory's notion that knowledge is valid regardless of the source. Advocates of this theory argue that good educational practice demands a more holistic approach when serving adults than was historically applied to traditional-aged students. One of the fundamental characteristics that distinguish adult learners from traditional college students is the years of experience they bring to a learning situation (Merriam and Caffarella, 1999). Many educators have considered this to be one of the most important distinctions between traditional and non-traditional students. Current cognitive, humanistic and constructivists learning models stress the importance of meaning-making (Merriam, Caffarella, and Baumgartner, 2012). Learning is viewed as an active process where an individual takes an idea or concept or problem and makes it their own by integrating the new learning with their own knowledge and experience. There has been an increased recognition by adult higher educators that the need to make sense of one's life experiences and what one knows can serve as an incentive for adults to engage in learning activities. The reflection and assessment of past experiences and prior knowledge has served as a motivator for adult learners to build upon prior learning, as well as enhancing the knowledge, skills and abilities they possess.

METHODS

Table 5.1 lists the different programmes typically associated with each prior learning assessment method and the organization(s) typically associated with overseeing each of the programmes.

TABLE 5.1 **Different Programmes and Sponsors Typically Associated with Each Prior Learning Assessment Category**

Category	Programme	Sponsor
Examination External	Advance Placement (AP) Examination Programme College Level Examination Programme (CLEP)	The College Board
	Defense Activity for Non-Traditional Education Support (DSST)	The Chauncey Group, a subsidiary of the Educational Testing Services
Internal	College and university challenge examination programmes (e.g. Excelsior University, Ohio University)	Colleges and Universities
Programme Evaluation	American Council on Education's Military	American Council on Education
	American Council on Education's College Credit Recommendation Services (ACE/CREDIT)	American Council on Education
Individualized approaches	Oral interviews Comprehensive demonstrations Portfolios	Colleges and universities

Testing is still the method most used by the institutions to award credit (CAEL, 2010). Two categories of examinations are used to evaluate prior learning: external, standardized examinations and internal, proficiency/challenge examinations. Standardized tests have been developed and marketed by such groups as the Educational Testing Services (ETS) and the American College Testing (ACT) in a variety of different subject areas. A committee of experts prepares the examinations, and test results are compared against traditional college courses to develop normative scores. In addition to external examination programmes, college and university faculty also prepare examinations for their own courses that students can challenge to receive credit. These examinations expand the subject areas available to students, and enables individual faculty to be more directly involved in both the preparation of the test and the evaluation of the individual learner.

As previously discussed, the American Council on Education (ACE) has evaluated military training and published college credit recommendations for colleges and universities to consider for awarding credit for learning from military training and experience. In 1974, ACE expanded this process to include the evaluations of on-going training programmes to any organization under the auspices of their College Credit Recommendation Services (ACE/CREDIT). ACE evaluations are conducted by teams of subject-matter experts drawn from a variety of post-secondary institutions. The variables used to determine college credit are the intended learning outcomes, the length of time, the levels of complexity and the methods to evaluate the participant's achievement of the learning outcomes. Credit recommendations are up-dated on a regular basis and results are accessible at the American Council on Education's website (www.acenet.edu). About 600 corporations, professional associates, labour unions and governmental agencies have used ACE/CREDIT services, ranging from Starbucks and McDonalds to the Federal Aviation Administration and the National Security Agency.

While important assessment tools, there are some inherent limitations with these two methods. Neither method provides a mechanism to assist individuals with the process of identifying and evaluating their own learning or how to develop a plan to enhance or build upon previous knowledge. An individual's prior learning is not always easily categorized into a traditional subject area, thus standardized tests may not be available. The prospect of testing makes many adult learners very uncomfortable, and merely offering a test does not address the issues of how to help adult learners know what test to take or how these tests relate to their career and academic goals. ACE programme evaluations have limited utility for the individual student interested in prior learning assessment; not all students have been in the military or participated in a programme evaluated by ACE.

A portfolio is the formal document that details learning acquired through non-college experiences. The document is used to request college recognition for the learning from experience. Typically, a portfolio includes the following parts: autobiographical information, goals statement, description of learning detailing an individual's request for college credit and documentation to support the learning. Faculty determines if the learning is equivalent to college-level learning and the amount of credit to award. The portfolio process offers both methodological and educational advantages over the other two methods. Many institutions provide a workshop or course to guide students through the process. Advising and assisting the learner to identify college-level learning and how such learning relates to the students overall degree plan are crucial components of a portfolio process. Preparation of the portfolio requires that learners develop a working model of their own learning process, expand their understanding of how they construct their world view and improve their self-directed learning skills, applying all of this to the completion of their lifelong learning goals (Sheckley and Keeton, 1995). Standardized tests, oral interviews, performance assessment and programme evaluations (ACE) are often incorporated into the portfolio process, allowing individuals to take advantage of all three methods.

IMPACT

The most basic question regarding assessment of prior learning is asked by both students and faculty. Is it worth the effort? Developing a portfolio is a complex task, requiring students to review their experiences, extract the learning and articulate the learning in a form that faculty can evaluate for college credit. When presented with the alternative of taking a class that is a repetition of prior learning, thousands of students have chosen prior learning assessment. Students are attracted to institutions with prior learning programmes, and they stay to complete their degrees at those institutions. CAEL's 2010 research study of 62,475 students at 48 post-secondary institutions supports this finding; students involved in the assessment of prior learning had much higher degree completion rates than adult learners who followed a more traditional route (CAEL, 2010). In addition to the academic recognition, the process helps students set realistic goals and develop educational plans. Students understand their level of expertise and how it relates to their degree plans, developing a broader understanding of educational requirements. Students' self-esteem increases as they receive validation of their learning experiences from prior experience.

Business and industry are attracted to institutions with prior learning assessment programmes because they view such programmes as a benefit for their employees and as a means to encourage employees to pursue academic degrees. The initial contact has created partnerships in other areas between the two groups to the benefit of both. An educated workforce is considered a necessity to remain competitive in today's world.

Institutions have found that creating an assessment of prior learning programme has assisted faculty to improve their classroom teaching because they must clearly articulate their expectations and articulation of learning outcomes for courses to facilitate the assessment of prior learning. The basic tenets of PLA challenge the traditional views of the instructional paradigm, challenging many faculty and administrators' assumptions about the teaching and learning process. This has served as an important catalyst for faculty to embrace the learning paradigm. Prior learning assessment requires that faculty be actively involved in the process and committed to assisting the learner. Faculty must examine their philosophy of learning and often refocus on their primary task, the learner. Procedures must be developed to guide students through the entire process; faculty input is essential for each step. Faculty must develop criterion standards, detailing what they mean by college-level learning to assist students as they prepare portfolios, as well as guide the evaluation of the portfolios. Evaluation of prior learning must be conducted by the faculty, addressing issues that affect reliability and validity. Organized portfolios assist faculty with the task of assessing prior learning. Educators actively involved in the assessment of prior learning argue that it is more than a method or set of practices for granting credit; it is a creative and critical process that leads to a critical reassessment of existing views of teaching and learning. Faculties involved in PLA have found that the process serves as a vehicle for learners to integrate theory with practice and for promoting reflective learning through the identification of learning from experience. Prior learning assessment can create an exciting partnership between faculty and students that can result in a interweaving of the world of work and the world of school.

Over the years many adult learners have benefited from the assessment of prior learning and there are a number of institutions that have developed comprehensive programmes for adult learners. However, not everyone in the higher education field has embraced the concept of prior learning assessment. Many educators still considered the concept a controversial issue. It is estimated that only half of the colleges and universities in the US accept some form of prior learning credit (Fain, 2012). The more selective colleges and universities with large number of traditional age students are often not willing to consider college credits based on prior learning assessment. The basic tenet that college-level learning can occur outside of a post-secondary institution's sponsorship has been a difficult idea for many faculty and administrators to embrace. Programme abuses, shoddy practices and lack of understanding have made many faculty members leery of the entire process. However there are some institutions that have been involved for many years. Almost 66 per cent of the 48 institutions CAEL surveyed in 2010 have offered PLA since the early 80s. They found that the institutions surveyed offered a range of PLA options with standardized exams (94 per cent) being the most common method used to assess prior learning. The majority of institutions offered multiple methods; 84 per cent offered four or more methods and 88 per cent of the institutions surveyed offered portfolio assessments. Hart and Hickerson's publication provides detailed description of 11 comprehensive programmes applying CAEL's standards of good practice (Hart and Hickerson, 2009).

A number of educators feel that low profile that prior learning assessment has experienced in the past is about to change as a result of the push for increasing college completion rates, the increase in the adult student market and the focus on continuous learning (Fain, 2012). CAEL and ACE will be major players in this movement; as early adopters in this arena they have set standards, policies and procedures for academic credible prior learning assessment programmes. ACE has decades of experience as well as a large network of faculty credit evaluators. CAEL recently introduced a new prior learning service, Learning Counts. They are offering a course to assist learners with the identification of prior learning and preparation of a portfolio. Working with ACE, faculty will be selected to evaluate the portfolios. A number of colleges and universities have agreed to send their students through the process and accept the credit recommendations from the Learning Counts programme; currently 150 institutions are participating in this programme (Learning Counts, 2012). Policy makers in several states are pushing prior learning assessment as an important part of the agenda to improve college completion rates. One in five Americans of working age has some college credit but no degree according in the Lumina Foundation (CAEL, 2010). Recognition of credit for prior learning can serve as a powerful motivator to complete degrees for these adults and reduce the time spent. Both proponents and critics argue for the need to ensure academic integrity in the design of prior learning programmes even more so with the increase pressure to offer this service to adult learners. With the increasing focus placed on PLA, abuses and high profile missteps could attract more attention and undermine the practice.

DESIGN OF PRIOR LEARNING ASSESSMENT PROGRAMMES

Over the years colleges and universities have developed a variety of ways to provide this service to adult learners, ranging from the development of policies regarding the various methods to comprehensive programmes Strong programmes have kept three obligations in mind as they have designed programme components: (1) a rationale that is consistent with the institution's mission and resources, (2) clearly articulated policies and procedures that are published for students and faculty and (3) consistent and fair implementation of policies and procedures (Fiddler and Marienau, 2009).

As stated, colleges and universities have made prior learning assessment available to adult learners in a variety of ways. Some institutions have simply developed policies and listed the policies in their catalogues. While this is an important process, it assumes that adult learners will locate the information and follow-thru on the process. The majority of adult learners need more assistance with the process of identifying what they have learned and how the learning matches with college courses. Responsibility for implementation of the policies is often housed in Registration offices which has little advising contact with learners. Overall this approach has resulted in little use of the assessment of prior learning with the exception of the evaluation of military transcripts using the ACE credit recommendations.

To provide better assistance to the adult learner numerous colleges and universities have developed workshops and/or courses to assist learners with the process of identify learning and how to develop a portfolio to serve as the assessment tool. Hart and Hickerson's publication describes how several institutions have organized their prior learning assessment programmes and includes examples of portfolios prepared by learners and results of their assessment (Hart and Hickerson, 2009). CAEL's 2010 research study found that the greater the flexibly the student has for using PLA credits, the better the academic outcomes. They explored 48 institutions that used PLA credits for advanced standing, to waive course pre-requisites, meet general education requirements and/or meet programme major requirements.

This finding was also supported in an earlier CAEL project to identify the best practices of an adult friendly institution (Flint, 1999). Stronger more effective programmes are programmes that actively integrated prior learning with the identification and completion of the learners' academic goals. Even when learners have had a great deal of experience with postsecondary institutions, they rarely understand how to best use all the resources the academy has to offer; finding higher learning a mysterious institution difficult to enter and exit in a meaningful way. The starting point begins with assisting the adult learner to clearly articulate their career and life goals and identify the academic programme that would help them accomplish these goals in an efficient and effective manner. From there learners explore their learning from experience, as well as previous educational experiences. It is not unusual for an adult learner to have accumulated college credits from more than one postsecondary institution. The development of the learner's educational plan is to create a pathway to accomplish their academic goals, building upon previous college courses and their prior learning. The development of the educational plan requires that the learner answer the following questions:

- What degree should I pursue?
- What specific courses do I need to complete for this degree?
- What courses will transfer from previous institutions to fulfil course requirements?
- How will my prior learning experiences assist me in completing the degree?
- What prior learning assessment options are available and how can I use them to fulfil course requirements?
- What is the best method given both the faculty and the learner's preferences and the subject matter?
- What courses am I going to have to complete and what options are available to me?

The last part of the process is to map out the detailed pathway with target dates for completion.

Figure 5.1 graphically articulates a very deliberate process to move the adult learner toward the completion of an academic goal. Learners are actively involved in the entire process; exploring options that best fit their unique situation. The educational institution has intentionally planned programmes and services to help learners move through the process. The learner learns about all the different methods to assess their prior learning and how to select those methods that fits their individual learning needs and preferences. The vast majority of adults need assistance in the identification of their learning from experience and how these learning outcomes match with college-level learning. This part of the advising process is crucial to successful programme participation and retention of adult learners. In addition the learner examines potential barriers to their success and ways to overcome the barriers. Too often due to work and family responsibilities adult learners must stop in and out of the academy; this integrated education plan serves as an important blueprint.

FIGURE 5.1 Process to move the adult learner toward the completion of an academic goal.

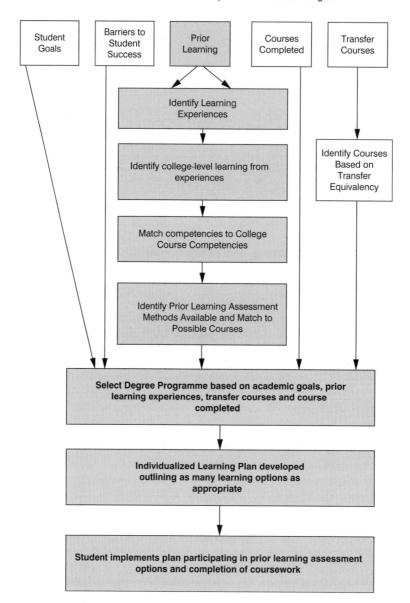

ADULT LEARNER EXAMPLE

Susan has reached a point in her career where her credentials are not enabling her to advance. She has over 20 years' experience in the health care field and would like to move from direct nursing care and counselling to administration. While she has some experience as a programme administrator she is finding that it is not sufficient as she explores positions as director of an assisted living facility for people 55 and older. After much research, she feels that a post-secondary degree combined with her experience would make her more desirable in the job market. She earned her nursing degree from an area hospital's nursing school. Upon passing her state boards she was employed for five years as a pulmonary intensive care nurse. From there she transferred to the Psychiatric Department for four years. As a result of her husband's job relocation, Susan changed jobs and worked as a school nurse for two years. She created and managed a programme overseeing the nurses at all the schools in the district for another four years. She created educational programmes for teens and their parents about substance abuse. Due to the success of the programme, she made numerous presentations about programme design and implementation. She then moved to a social service agency counselling youth and adults about substance abuse as assistant director. She quickly advanced at this agency expanding her experiences and knowledge in administration, grant-writing and programme evaluation. After five years, the agency funding was drastically reduced and Susan found it necessary to re-enter the job market. Throughout her career she took advantage of educational opportunities that were made available to her. She has taken several continuing education courses in the health care field, counselling, management and programme funding. She has also taken several courses at the local community college. In addition to her work experience Susan has been active in her church where she has created educational programmes for the teenagers. She served on the church council in a number of different capacities and worked closely with a team to raise the funds and build a new church. She was actively involved in the building design and the construction phase.

After exploring the job market Susan feels that a post-secondary degree would make her more desirable in the job market. While she enjoyed the direct patient care and education, she loves the challenge of administration and helping an organization grow and develop to serve a larger constituency. At the age of 43, she is not quite sure how to get started; she knows she does not want to completely start at the beginning to earning an academic degree. She feels strongly that her prior work experience has taught her a great deal and she would like to build upon her prior learning. After exploring several post-secondary institutions Susan enrolled in a college that had a programme designed for adult learners. She chose the college because they offered degrees in health care administration and gerontology along with the ability to participate in the assessment of her prior learning. The college also offered courses in a variety of different formats which would allow Susan to juggle work and family responsibilities to complete her degree.

The first course that Susan took was the school's Prior Learning Assessment Course. Working with the course instructor and faculty advisor, Susan decided that the Health Care Administration degree programme would be the best choice given her career goals and her prior learning. She had a transcript from the community college sent to the college and her advisor mapped out how the courses would apply to the Health Care Administration degree. Once she understood all the prior learning options that were available to her, Susan identified the courses and the methods she planned to use. Using all the information she had collected, Susan developed the following educational plan.

EDUCATIONAL PLANNING WORKSHEET
DEGREE PROGRAMME: HEALTH CARE ADMINISTRATION

Prior Learning Courses	Portfolio	Proficiency Exam	CLEP/DANTES	ACE/CREDIT	ACE Military	Projected Completion Date	New Learning Courses Completed	X	To Be Completed	Instructional Method	Projected Completion Date
English Composition			X				Accounting	X	Budgeting and Forecasting	C[1]	
Public Speaking	X						Introduction to Religion	X	Managerial Accounting	C	
Principles of Management	X						Economics	X	Project Management	O	
Computer Applications in Business		X					Foundation of Business	X	Health Service Information System	O	
Substance Abuse	X						Psychology	X	Health Service Finance	C	
Intro the Health Services	X								Managerial Care and Health Insurance	O	
Health Care Rights and Responsibilities	X								College Algebra	C	
Biology			X						Statistics for Business	C	
Sociology			X						Senior Project	I	
Health Care and Marketing	X								Intro to Gerontology	I	
Business Communications	X										

[1] C Classroom, O distance learning , I independent study

Susan found her experiences at this institution much different than the two other times she tried to return to school. She has a much broader understanding of the entire process having researched the Health Care Administration degree programme in its entirety and examined how fits together as a whole. She understands the programme outcomes and the courses that will help her meet those outcomes. She has explored the available PLA options and selected the courses she plans to challenge, as well as the methods she will use. Working with her advisors and faculty she has developed a plan that is both efficient and effective. She is excited to get started, confident that she has a blueprint for success.

KEY LEARNING ACTIVITY 16

The following learning activity can be used with an individual learner or as the one of the beginning steps in assessing how well your institution meets the needs of adult learners.

Use the following questions and the Educational Planning Worksheet and explore how you can assist an adult learner at your institution.

What degree should I pursue?

What specific courses do I need to complete for this degree?

What courses will transfer from previous institutions to fulfil course requirements?

How will my prior learning experiences assist me in completing the degree?

What prior learning assessment options are available and how can I use them to fulfil course requirements? What is the best method given both the faculty and the learner's preferences and the subject matter?

What courses am I going to have to complete and what options are available to me?

EDUCATIONAL PLANNING WORKSHEET
DEGREE PROGRAMME:

Prior Learning Courses	Portfolio	Proficiency Exam	CLEP/DANTES	ACE/CREDIT	ACE Military	Projected Completion Date	New Learning Courses Completed	Transfer Credit To Be Completed	Instructional Method	Projected Completion Date

For a learner – Use the information collected and the worksheet to finalize your plans for completing your academic goals.

For an institutional assessment tool – use this information to identify how comprehensive your services are for adult learners:

How does your institution guide adult learners through the process?

Are the policies and procedures documented and readily available for students to access? Who is responsible?

How involved are faculty with the process?

What are our priorities? What changes are needed to better serve adult learners?

What are the gaps in your services?

The information from this activity can serve as a starting point to assess how to improve on the ways your institution serves adult learners.

SUMMARY

The aim of this chapter has been to provide an overview of prior learning assessment in the United States. It has explored the historical development and the impact of prior learning assessment on adult learners. The reasons for the growth of prior learning assessment were presented, along with the primary methods employed to assess prior learning. Finally, the Chapter discussed the importance of educational planning and an integrated approach necessary to assist adult learners in completing their academic goals.

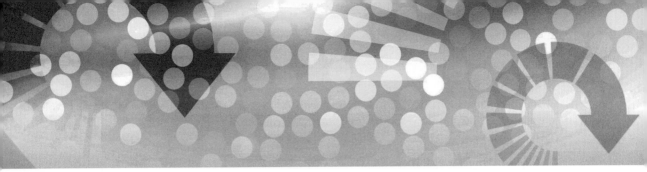

CHAPTER 6
THE CASE OF A
HUMAN SERVICES
RELATED PROGRAMME
IN MAURITIUS

This Chapter offers a detailed analysis of the Mauritian model for RPL. It highlights the factors which triggered the implementation of RPL within the Mauritian Education and Training system and its impact on the growth of the individual.

This Chapter will also elaborate on the key players within the process and evolution of RPL in Mauritius while identifying the difficulties and tensions which have underpinned the establishment and development of RPL within the Mauritian context. Finally it will discuss the issues which have been identified post the implementation phase.

At the end of this Chapter, the reader will be able to:

● Provide an overview of the key elements in the development of RPL in Mauritius.

● Describe the methodology adopted by the Mauritius Qualifications Authority in the establishment of RPL.

● Identify variations in the Mauritian RPL Model.

● Identify the challenges underpinning implementation of RPL in Mauritius.

BACKGROUND

Before embarking on discussions relating to RPL practice in Mauritius, it is important to trace back its evolution and the context in which RPL was introduced within the education and training system.

Socio-economic characteristic

Situated in the Indian Ocean, the islands of Mauritius are of volcanic origin and consist of the main island of Mauritius, Rodrigues and two smaller groups of islands. Once reliant on the cultivation of sugar cane as the foundation of its growth strategy, the island suffered at the turn of millennium when hit by the removal of the European trade preference after having benefited for over 40 years under the Sugar Protocol of the Lomé Conventions. The Government had to review its Strategic Planning in order to adapt itself to a new culture of fast-changing societal landscapes. Change was inevitable and the Mauritian Government multiplied its efforts towards market diversification to include Tourism, Financial Services, the Real Estate sector, the Information and Communication Technology (ICT) sector and the Seafood Hub. Following a successful transformation from a low-income, agriculture-based economy to a diversified upper middle-income economy, the socio-economic conditions of the Island was gradually stabilized.

However, with the changes taking place, the Government acknowledged the need to re-train and up-skill its manpower in order to achieve a competitive human capital and better arm itself to face major challenges within its economy both at the local and international level. It became evident that Mauritius was facing difficulties with respect to increasing mismatch in labour skills, jobs as well as scarce human resource capabilities in certain economic sectors. Concurrently, the economic crisis undoubtedly led to the marginalization of those having work experience but no formal qualification. For example, with new sectors emerging a void had been created for those working within sectors in decline such as the Sugar and Textile Industry (The percentage of those falling out of the system is underlined in Table 6.1 below). Therefore, there was a clear need to prepare for a productive, flexible workforce crucial to competition in the 21st century, which implied restructuring the Mauritian economic base.

In addition, as per the statistics of the Mauritius Examinations Syndicate nearly 31.44 per cent fail at the CPE examinations. The Government had already taken specific measures for those failing to integrate the system by channelling them into the pre-vocational stream for three years with the aim to join the vocational sector by enrolling onto National Certificates, as highlighted on the right side of Figure 6.1. However, the Mauritian education and training system has recently witnessed more changes. With increasing emphasis being made on LLL, the Government has reviewed the pre-vocational stream from three years to four with learners being awarded the Level 1 National Certificates rather than the National Trade Certificate (NTC) Foundation award. Other reforms are also being implemented towards the integration of people having no formal qualifications but having gained experience. For instance, a large percentage of those falling out of the system quickly find themselves assimilated within the world of work. Though failing to integrate the academic stream many of them become apt skilled workers learning on the job and through experience. The necessity to have such experience and training recognized is undoubtedly vital for such persons.

In fact, countries around the world are witnessing a gradual change in the qualifications system regimes. The need to have qualifications which meet contemporary developments in the labour market brought governments across the world to review and re-structure their education and training systems. Having acknowledged the role of education, training and qualifications, Mauritius in turn established the National Qualification Framework (NQF) to attain greater qualifications coverage and offer more pathway linkages so as to motivate Mauritians to embark on education and training pathways. Placed under the guardianship of the Mauritius Qualifications Authority (MQA), the NQF reinforces progression routes, enhancing the possibilities to have more qualifications and rendering it more flexible to adapt itself to the changing demands of the labour market.

TABLE 6.1 Labour Force, Employment and Unemployment, 16 Years and Over, 2001–2009 (Note that the Figures are in '000)

Year	Labour Force			Employment including foreign workers			Unemployment	
	Mauritian	Foreign Workers	Total	in large establish-ments[1]	outside large establish-ments	Total	Number	Rate[2] (%)
Both sexes								
2001	510.3	16.5	526.8	302.0	190.1	492.1	34.7	6.8
2002	513.0[3]	17.0	530.0	297.2	196.0	493.2	36.8	7.2
2003	520.9	18.2	539.1	296.9	202.1	499.0	40.1	7.7
2004	531.3	17.5	548.8	293.3	210.9	504.2	44.6	8.4
2005	542.5	16.6	559.1	292.2	215.0	507.2	51.9	9.6
2006	548.4	16.7	565.1	295.1	220.2	515.3	49.8	9.1
2007	548.9	21.6	570.5	302.0	221.7	523.7	46.8	8.5
2008	559.4	24.0	583.4	311.6	231.4	543.0	40.4	7.2
2009	566.3	21.0	587.3	306.0	239.8	545.8	41.5	7.3

[1]Employing ten or more persons
[2]Unemployment as a percentage of Mauritian labour force
[3]The low increase results from the implementation of the Voluntary Retirement Scheme (VRS) in the sugar industry
Source: (Central Statistics Office, *Digest of Education Statistics 2010*)

Establishment of RPL

Led by this new wave of revolution, the concept of Recognition of Prior Learning (RPL) was evoked in the Mauritian context. The necessity to reconcile existing skills with the demands for new skills and new trends culminated in the establishment of RPL within the education and training system so as to cater for those who were being left out of the system and to maintain a competitive and skilled workforce. The quality of education and training on offer and the notion of lifelong learning had already been identified as key factors in the continued development of the country given that they better equip the human capital to adapt and evolve in emerging economic sectors and also the social development of individuals. Using the NQF as its foundation and being empowered by the MQA Act 2001 'to recognise and validate competencies for the purpose of certification obtained outside the formal education and training systems', MQA formally introduced RPL in the Mauritian system in response to the changing demographics of the Mauritian economy by directly tackling the issue of up-skilling/retraining of its workforce while acknowledging their existing skills. In short RPL, acting as a mechanism for inclusion, offers greater access to individuals by validating their knowledge and skills, arising from any kind of learning environment and unrelated to the academic context. By combining and building on learning achieved people can thus be rewarded for it via National Certificates, allowing them to move within the labour market better equipped.

Much of this non-formal or informal learning is relevant to the competency outcomes of Unit Standards as developed by the MQA and can subsequently be pitched on the Mauritian NQF given that awarding

FIGURE 6.1   The Current structure of the Mauritian Education and Training System

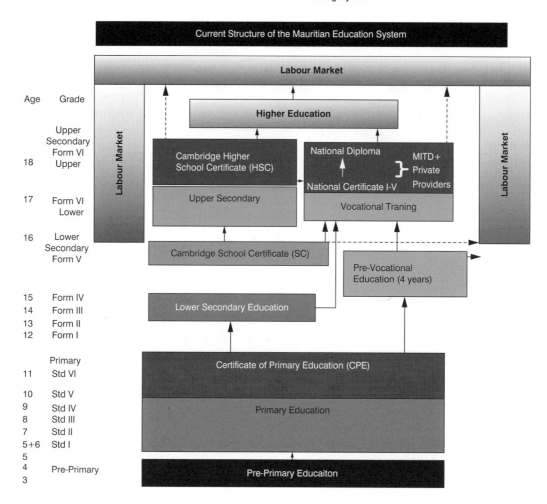

bodies use the Unit Standards to develop evaluation grids which are needed in building the Portfolio and assessment for RPL. For example, a person having worked in the Tourism Industry for 12 years may have his/her experiences assessed against the outcomes of the Unit Standards (See Figure 6.2 for further details). The main focus of RPL is therefore the learning outcomes, in the form of skills and knowledge of experiences, and not how, when and where the learning occurred. As such RPL helps to bring people back to education and training systems and allows them to progress within the NQF by acquiring a duly recognized national qualification. RPL is thus seen as a critical aspect in the implementation of the NQF.

Acting as a feeder to further and higher education, RPL thereby helps expand educational and employment opportunities for the individual. Consequently helping to increase the Gross Enrolment Ratio at Tertiary level, which in turn alleviates poverty as people can get better jobs. Therefore RPL contributes to the social and economic development of the nation. More importantly, this new system assists in reducing the number of illiterate people and encourages people to pursue further with their studies.

FIGURE 6.2 Re-integration into the system through RPL

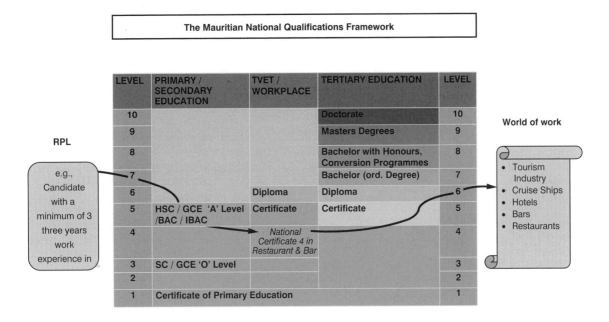

KEY LEARNING ACTIVITY 17

1   After having reviewed the Background of this Chapter identify the opportunities and benefits of implementing RPL in the Mauritian Education and Training System.

2   Do you believe that the RPL system is based on the 'one size fits all' approach?

THE MAURITIAN RPL MODEL

Methodology adopted

Prior to the implementation of RPL in Mauritius, the MQA proceeded with a qualitative research which consisted mainly of a literature and desk research conducted via documentation review and an international workshop with various national stakeholders and international interlocutors with the aim to ascertain the relevancy of RPL in Mauritius. However, despite the fact that the concept of RPL was not new to the academic sphere, and had already been implemented by Governments across continents, some difficulty was experienced as RPL was being employed in higher education sectors rather than the TVET sector specifically. In fact, RPL was traced back as far as 1792 (Pouget and Osborne, 2004) in the French history in the context of '*formation continue*' (lifelong learning) and to the 1940s in USA with the evaluation of the skills of soldiers returning from war for recognition by universities (Andersson and Harris, 2006). After considerable efforts, the data on the systems and procedures adopted by different countries were taken into consideration and analyzed. A comparative analysis was carried out to examine the varying RPL models being used. To this end, the structures adopted within the following countries were used as research sample: South Africa, Scotland, Australia, Canada, France and England (See Table 6.2).

It became evident that RPL had many roots some leading to discussions regarding experiential learning while others led to the concept of lifelong learning or social justice where it was perceived as a means of economic integration and social inclusion. Yet, in spite of being differently defined, there was a common thread in between all the definitions, that is, the recognition of previous experience, skills, knowledge and informal learning. As such, while the essence of RPL remained the same, it was moulded to suit the demographic, technological and economic landscapes of the island.

However, regardless of the terminology used, RPL was identified as a form of assessment, a holistic approach where both the social and the learning context of the learner were taken into consideration. This approach avoided the assessment from becoming a purely technical application. Recognition of prior learning builds on the basic notion that the individual should not learn the same thing twice but should have the opportunity to use and build on his or her competences, irrespective of where and how they were acquired.

TABLE 6.2 Variation in Appellation of Prior Learning

Country	Appellation	Definition
South Africa	Recognition of Prior Learning – RPL	Recognition of prior learning means the comparison of the previous learning and experience of a learner howsoever obtained against the learning outcomes required for a specified qualification, and the acceptance for purposes of qualification of that which meets the requirement.
Scotland	Accreditation of Prior (Experiential) Learning – APL/ APEL	Accreditation of Prior Learning, the process which enables candidates to receive certification for past achievements. These may have been acquired through work experience, leisure pursuits or training. APL focuses on the competences which can be demonstrated at the time.
Australia	Recognition of Prior Learning – RPL	RPL involves the assessment of previously unrecognized skills and knowledge an individual has achieved outside the formal education and training system.
Canada	Prior Learning Assessment and Recognition – PLAR	Prior Learning Assessment and Recognition is a process that recognizes adult learning connected to experiential learning and how it can be articulated against academic credit or industry standards.
France	Validation des Acquis d'Expérience – VAE	The VAE process enables an individual to get a full or part certification based on his/her professional experience (salaried, non-salaried or voluntary).
England	Accreditation of Prior Experiential Learning – APEL	Accreditation of Prior And Experiential Learning (APEL) is a process that enables people of all ages, backgrounds and attitudes to receive formal recognition for skills and knowledge they already possess.

Based on the above, the Mauritian RPL model was formulated and subsequently major stakeholders were exposed to international best practises of RPL and its benefits towards the economic growth of the island.

The benefits of RPL

RPL was seen to offer an array of benefits to Mauritians, that is, the learners, employers and the Nation. While it helps individual learners:

a) to ease the transition from informal and non-formal to formal learning by enabling the learners to value their achievements and to recognize the importance of their learning through experience;

b) to plan for further learning and personal/career development;

c) to gain entry to a programme of study (if they do not have the normal entry qualifications);

d) to obtain credit towards a programme of study thereby shortening the period of study.

RPL can support training and staff development strategies of employers by:

a) Increasing motivation and interest in workplace practice on the part of the employee/learner.

b) Reducing the amount of time needed to complete a qualification and therefore requiring less time away from the workplace.

c) Improving employee retention and preventing duplication of training.

Subsequently, the country benefits by:

● Having a certified skilled workforce.

● Having an empowered and multi-skilled population.

● Attracting investors to position Mauritius in the global village.

● Reducing the cost of training of people.

● Having an efficient response to industry skill shortages.

Following a positive response from stakeholders MQA set about the development of RPL. The task at hand was to develop a model where non-academic learning would be translated onto the education and training system. Thus an adaptation of the French RPL, that is, *Validation des Acquis d'Expérience* commonly known as VAE, was envisaged. However, it was deemed that the term '*Recognition of Prior Learning*' was more apt for the Mauritian context given it could encompass both formal and informal learning. In its endeavour to launch RPL, MQA was assisted by the Commonwealth of Learning (COL) and the UNESCO Institute for Lifelong Learning (UIL) and L'Academié de La Reunion. In the first instance, the MQA collaborated with COL to organize an international workshop on RPL so as to expose major stakeholders to international RPL best practices and provide insights into the various advantages linked to the implementation of RPL at a national level. And given the expertise of the UIL and L'Academié de La Reunion in the domain of RPL, their collaboration was sought for the development of the Mauritian RPL policy as well as capacity building and training of MQA staff, facilitators and assessors respectively. Various workshops were organized to this end. The aim of these exercises being:

● To define RPL and the RPL process.

● To judge the suitability of RPL candidates.

● To explain the RPL evidence requirements.

● How to help candidates in portfolio development while remaining neutral.

● How to facilitate the RPL.

● To train assessors in the conduct of RPL assessments process.

● To inform assessors of the core principles of the NQF and RPL.

In order for the potential of RPL to be realized, it was evident that the collaboration between institutions, that is national stakeholders as well as international institutions, would be necessitated. Despite having the structure in place, without the acceptance or involvement of national stakeholders sustaining RPL becomes an even more challenging task. As such consolidating networks not only safeguards RPL but is crucial to its evolution.

The process

Reflecting on international norms, the Mauritian RPL is a three-stage process (see Figure 6.3 below), comprising of the Pre-Screening Process, the Facilitation Process and the Assessment Process. Each stage is closely monitored by the MQA, beginning with stage 1 where MQA carries out the pre-screening process and thereafter overseeing the facilitation process. To further promote transparency assessment is carried out independently by a competent Awarding Body. The three stages are designed to ensure that the process is quality assured to protect the integrity of the mechanism. The aims of the RPL process (shown in Figure 6.3) are as follows:

a) Identify what the learner knows and can do.

b) Match the skills, knowledge and experience of the learner with the unit standards as developed by the MQA.

c) Assess the learner.

d) Acknowledge the competencies of the learner.

e) Credit the learner for skills, knowledge and experience already acquired through assessment.

f) Issue of a record of learning (part qualification)/ full qualification.

Figure 6.3 offers the schema of the 3 main stages of the Mauritian RPL process as conceived by the MQA.

FIGURE 6.3 The RPL Process

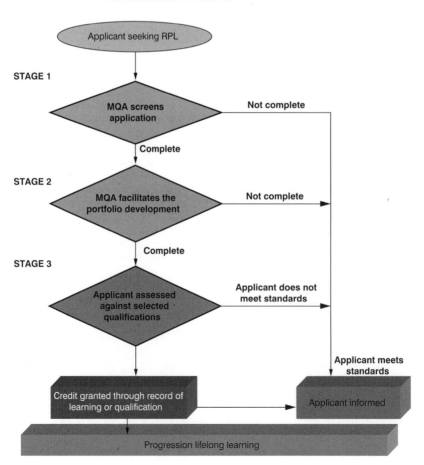

Other than institutional key players within the RPL process, the role of Staff within MQA, Facilitators and Assessors, that is, those who are in direct contact with the candidates are equally important. In fact the quality of RPL depends significantly on the approach adopted by the above mentioned people. Continuous training for the staff, facilitators and institutions involved in the process not only ensures reliability but safeguards RPL practices.

Stage 1 – The pre-screening process provides the applicant with all services and support in terms of advice and counselling. The latter is fully informed of the application process, the stages within the RPL process and the portfolio development. The MQA staff ensures that the potential applicant is eligible for claiming RPL and has selected the appropriate qualification. The initial contact is very crucial to the applicant since the latter is informed about the principles behind RPL, the procedures, the cost implication and mounting of the portfolio which ensures that the candidate adequately transfers his/her experience onto paper.

Stage 2 – The RPL Facilitator is the second key contact of the applicant. The first meeting is carried out by MQA but it is the Facilitator who guides and supports the applicant in developing the Portfolio of evidences. More precisely, the facilitator helps and advises the applicant on the necessary evidences that should be submitted or any missing information or documents that are related to the applicant's portfolio. In short, the Facilitator facilitates the transition between non-formal and formal learning contexts and identifies core skills gained informally which can be transferred to formal learning contexts in various contexts. The Facilitator should be well-versed with the Unit Standards and the learning demands given that the Facilitator provides guidance and ensures that the applicant has realistic expectations.

The MQA is subsequently responsible for the training as well as the registration of the RPL Facilitators. Appointed by the MQA, the Facilitator communicates to the learner the different options of building the portfolio by guiding the latter in the compilation of evidences in a coherent and systematic manner and spends a minimum of ten hours with the candidate over a period of three months. The duration of facilitation process is vital given that learners get sufficient time to reflect over their past experience before transcribing same on paper. Once the learner has met the requirements for recognition of the prior learning, the learner is subsequently guided towards the RPL assessment.

The Facilitator should:

(i)   Have strong communication abilities.

(ii) Have good interview skills.

(iii) Be able to make applicants reflect on experience to identify knowledge, skills, attitudes, behaviour, real life situations and experience in non-formal and informal contexts.

(iv) Be able to do notional levelling or mapping in relation to Unit Standards and Qualifications.

Unlike other countries, facilitators in Mauritius can only assist people within their field of competency unlike France where the facilitator can assist candidates from various sectors. The assessment consists of both formative and summative elements comprising a portfolio and an assessment which is conducted at the end of the process in the form of an interview.

Stage 3 – The third stage deals with the assessment process. The role of the assessor is to compare the applicant's evidences provided in the portfolio with the unit standards of the NQF qualification and to assess the competencies acquired. It is the assessor's responsibility to:

● use the criteria for assessment;

● use appropriate assessment techniques;

● ensure that the evidence provided is sufficient to make impartial judgements;

● record assessment results;

● provide detailed feedback to the applicant;

● ensure that assessment procedures are recorded correctly and all parties are advised;

● maintain the integrity of the assessment system;

● comply with assessment instructions provided by the Assessment Centre.

The training of RPL assessors is a critical component for the success of implementing the RPL procedure. The assessors need to be trained in accordance to prevailing norms as they have to show professional judgement in assessing the value of experience *vis à vis* formal learning. Training ensures that a holistic approach is maintained when dealing with learners, that is abiding to rules of transparency, reliability, validity, consistency and coherence while guiding the latter to build his/her portfolio.

All RPL assessments are carried out by nationally recognized awarding bodies. Successful applicants are issued either a part qualification or a full qualification at the end of the process. Qualifications issued to RPL candidates do not differ from those issued to candidates through formal examination. In case the applicant fails to meet the required standards, s/he is informed of same.

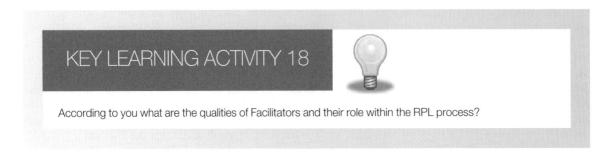

KEY LEARNING ACTIVITY 18

According to you what are the qualities of Facilitators and their role within the RPL process?

Enactment of awarding bodies for RPL

One of the critical steps in the implementation of RPL in Mauritius was the establishment of Awarding Bodies. As highlighted in Stage 3 of the RPL process, the culmination of the RPL process is carried out in the final stage where the candidate is assessed. In fact, in Mauritius, the Awarding Body is the entity responsible for the development of evaluation grids, on which the RPL assessment is based. Although the Awarding Bodies are not an integral part of the MQA, the authority is in close collaborations with the institutions to ensure the smooth process of RPL learners. Currently there are three major national institutions which have been identified as recognized awarding bodies; they are namely the Mauritius Institute of Training and Development (MITD) and Mauritius Institute of Health (MIH) for technical and vocational qualifications and the Mauritius Examinations Syndicate (MES). Having independent Awarding Bodies reinforce the continuous enhancement of quality and maintenance of the NQF. And though the role of the Mauritian NQF is undeniably to facilitate the inclusion of qualifications on the frameworkthe MQA is also fully committed to develop an educated and informed nation which shall act as a key driver in the development of the country. However compared to some other countries which transcribe RPL in the form of credits, the Mauritian candidates are awarded a duly recognized Certificate or a record of learning should they receive part qualification instead of a full qualification.

Development of the pilot projects

In view of the growing demand of the Tourism and Hospitality Sector within the Mauritian economy, the first pilot project was conducted so as to provide this booming industry with adequate, reliable and resilient employees. In addition, with the revolution in the economic sector and the number of people falling out of the education and training system, Mauritius had been witnessing a surge of skilled employees with no formal qualifications. RPL ensured that a second chance was given to such workers and disadvantaged groups, offering them the incentive to continue to learn and to become more active in the labour market.

Thus, with the financial collaboration of the Empowerment Programme[1] 30 volunteers were obtained for the RPL Pilot Project through the following institutions:

---

[1]The Empowerment Programme is part of the New Economic Agenda and has been implemented to democratize the economy by broadening the circle of opportunities to each Mauritian citizen, creating employment and bringing social justice, subsequently unlocking opportunities for the unemployed, for those recycled from their jobs, for women, for our young people entering the labour force and for small and medium entrepreneurs. The Programme also aimed to facilitate the transition from sugar, textiles and other activities hit by shocks, into higher value.

(i) L'Association des Hôteliers et Restaurateurs (AHRIM);

(ii) Mauritius Sugar Producers' Association through Highlands Sugar Estate; and

(iii) Virtual Centre for Innovative Learning Technologies (VCLIT) of University of Mauritius (List of unemployed persons).

These candidates were called for general information and briefed on RPL Procedures as well as the rationale of the RPL process. Most of the candidates belonged to working class backgrounds and had been excluded from academic education. The response was positive and a second meeting, in smaller groups, was carried out. Out of the 30 candidates, 25 pursued further with the pilot project and were assigned in the following fields of the Tourism and Hospitality sector: Housekeeping, Food Production, Pastry, Restaurant and Bar Services and Front Office. Following the first pilot project the policy was refined and stress was laid on the number of years a candidate was to have within the required field prior to applying for RPL in same. And more importantly, in addition to French and English, henceforth candidates were able to use the local language known as Creole to build their portfolios and during RPL assessment. Subsequently, the redefined policy was tested with a second pilot project in the Construction Industry. With the promising results obtained, in June 2009 MQA launched RPL in Mauritius in four trades, namely in Tourism, Construction, Printing and Plumbing. In 2010 RPL was extended to Adult Literacy and the following year it expanded to encompass Agriculture, Automotive Mechanics, Panel Beating and Spray Painting, Electrical Installation Works, Garment Making and Automotive Electricity and Electronics.

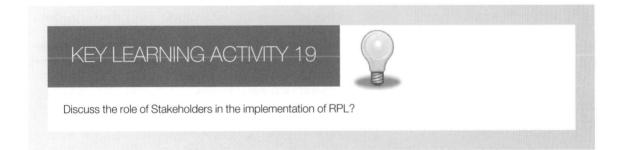

KEY LEARNING ACTIVITY 19

Discuss the role of Stakeholders in the implementation of RPL?

THE CURRENT STATUS

The successful implementation of RPL has substantially helped bridge the gap between lifelong learning and the existing skills of the workforce. With the structure formally in place, RPL candidates are now being awarded NQF qualifications through the certification system as established by the NQF. This initiative undoubtedly brings people back into the education and training system, subsequently providing Mauritius with a qualified labour force and paving the way for lifelong learning. With formal, informal and non-formal learning having been made official parts of the Mauritian Education and Training system, the culture for lifelong learning has been further enhanced. In the Mauritian Education and Human Resources Strategy Plan 2008–2020 the need: 'to create the conditions to enhance lifelong learning opportunities which include the recognition of prior learning and prior experiential learning … the development of multi-skilling and re-skilling programmes and the conduct of action research in the development of lifelong learning' have been clearly highlighted. Today, Mauritians have the possibility to climb up the social ladder by having their past experiences and skills validated. Mr Michael Sham an RPL Candidate in the Tourism Sector was awarded full RPL certificate in NTC Food Production Level 3. He stated that the certificate proved beneficial to him in that his work experience was officially recognized thus he gained more respect by his colleagues and also increased his chances for promotion, ultimately greater earning potential. Lifelong learning clearly goes beyond the education and training paradigm, encompassing the social as well as the cultural development of the individuals, that is, the personal growth of the individual. In addition, Mr Areff Salauroo, the President of the Mauritian Association of

Human Resource Professionals (AHRP), at its Annual General Meeting held on 30 April 2012 commended the RPL as developed by MQA as an effective and valuable tool for Human Resource Development and Management and 2012 also witnessed the expansion of RPL throughout all the technical and vocational sectors of the Mauritian economy.

Lessons learnt

From its inception to its implementation, innumerable lessons have been learnt with each step taken to establish RPL within the Mauritian education and training system. Some of the most pertinent issues faced are:

- **Capacity Building** – Given the nature and scope of work at hand, it became quickly apparent that there was a dearth of trained staff and facilitators. This void had to be urgently tackled so as to ensure the smooth establishment of the Mauritian RPL model and allowing clear diffusion of information to be passed on to the population.

- **Institutional Problems** – The absence of Technical and Vocational Education and Training (TVET) Awarding Bodies and as such appropriate infrastructures for assessment constituted another barrier. For instance, having no evaluation grids or set system to conduct assessment of National Certificates considerably hampered the assessment process as well as the enrolment of candidates onto RPL programmes. The need for a comprehensive and clear structure with well-defined purposes became apparent. Although the creation of the Mauritius Institute of Training and Development (MITD) filled the void of an awarding body in the TVET sector, being a new institution many issues were yet to be settled.

- **Lack of Critical mass for RPL** – RPL has undoubtedly brought changes to the existing education and training system, having introduced a new concept and with it a new mind-set and change in culture by formalizing prior learning undertaken in informal contexts. To ensure its success it is vital to communicate the ideologies behind RPL and its value to potential candidates and stakeholders. However, despite heavy campaigning and workshops being conducted, there has been a clear disinterest from the public to partake in RPL. Though trained, Facilitators have not come forth to be registered with MQA to facilitate RPL candidates, whereas the public has showed itself as being still sceptical of the concept of RPL.

- **Competition between formal routes of training and the process for RPL** – With more than 507 private training institutions offering training courses, RPL was at risk of being relegated by the population. Distinctions made between qualifications awarded through conventional and RPL routes had to be removed from the mind-set of people.

- **Time Constraint** – RPL clearly presupposed a strong National Qualifications Framework which is fully developed and expanding over various sectors. However, with National Qualifications still being developed, the task to expand RPL proved an even more challenging task which required time.

- **Misconceptions** – If some remained unconvinced by RPL, others embarked on it as an easy way out. Failing to understand the proceedings, applicants have tried to finish their portfolios earlier which resulted in the obtainment of part qualifications.

- **Quality Assurance Mechanisms** – Quality Assurance has to be under constant scrutiny. Effective measures to ensure the efficiency of the RPL system, i.e. Registration of Facilitators etc., have to be developed. The RPL policy will have to be revised and aligned to meet the changing demands and current market needs.

- **Cost** – The costing of the overall procedure has also been a deterring factor in the enrolment of candidates, who are mostly underprivileged. Although the cost of RPL is subsidized by the Government, through the funding being allocated to the MQA, applicants still face financial difficulties. Often self-employed, the situation is further complicated as they do not benefit from an employer's support. It is to be noted that the overall cost for RPL is currently 4300 Mauritian Rupees which is equivalent to 142 US Dollars.

Challenges

Despite Governmental and institutional commitment towards the implementation of RPL to widen access and render the system more flexible by acknowledging prior experiences, many barriers are still to be overcome. As highlighted in the lessons learnt, substantial challenges have been evoked which may hinder the proper functioning of RPL within the Mauritian context. Capacity building and the formalization of support infrastructures need to be consolidated and continually enhanced if progress is to be made. RPL is clearly not based on the premise that one size fits all but is moulded to reflect the changes taking place within the social and economic structure of the country. And more importantly to achieve its full potential as a transformative force within the education and training system, efforts have to be re-doubled so that the change being brought by RPL is accepted by institutions and people alike. The shift from institution-based and programme-based assessment to learner-based and competence-based assessment through RPL is a major challenge. This remains one of the main difficulties being faced by the MQA. The relationship with relevant stakeholders and institutions demand continual work to ensure effective progression.

Additionally, securing the trust of the public in the principles of Mauritian RPL model requires clear and concise information being communicated to the public. A culture shift is indispensible to allow greater value to be attached to vocational skills and to bring the formal education system and non-formal learning closer together. The task at hand is to maintain these relationships while consolidating the foundation of RPL to gain credibility within Mauritius. The need to raise awareness among stakeholders and the public had led to the organization of continuous sensitization campaigns across the island to reach out to the mass and raise awareness about RPL and its benefits. Informational Workshops are also constantly being organized for various stakeholders. The challenge that now lies ahead is the sustainability of the system, forging an enabling environment within the traditional education and training system of Mauritius which shall endorse the smooth integration of the RPL model.

So far, RPL has been tested and carried out on lower level qualifications but expanding to higher level qualifications, i.e. Diploma levels, still need to be formalized. It is evident that some aspects of the Mauritian RPL model have yet to be established. Benchmarks and a range of support mechanisms are essential for its progression.

Time is required for the above mentioned measure to have any true bearings. During the implementation process, from the key lessons learnt, one crucial element which became apparent is that RPL is not static but rather a dynamic process, where we have to learn from past experiences to better secure the future of RPL and its candidates. This demands time, effort and capital on behalf of the Mauritian Government to achieve its goal towards an enhanced education and training system which will be an umbrella of learning systems encompassing formal, informal and non-formal learning to promote lifelong learning.

SUMMARY

The aim of this Chapter has been to provide an overview of the implementation of RPL within the Education and Training system of Mauritius by the Mauritius Qualifications Authority, from the social to the economic aspects of its inception. It identified the key players involved in the conception of the mechanism and those involved in its structural foundation. Finally it also highlighted the challenges and tensions which have underpinned its establishment.

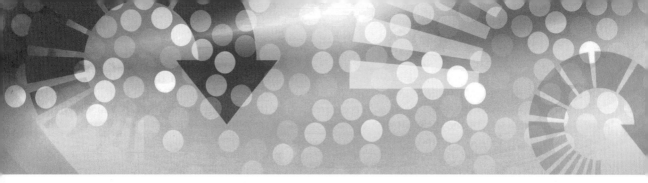

CHAPTER 7
THE CAREER OF THE
APL PRACTITIONER

Chapters 1 and 2 discussed how benchmarks for assessment of prior learning have been introduced to lend greater clarity to the assessment process. This Chapter will discuss in more detail how these benchmarks relate to the ongoing career of the APL practitioner and how they might be used to support the practitioner's continuing professional development.

At the end of this Chapter the reader will have explored:

- The theory of 'Career' as applied to the teaching professions.

- Identified the specific 'Career Path' of the APL practitioner.

- The holistic nature of prior learning assessment and implications of this for faculty.

- Identified how benchmarks for practice can be used to support the continuing professional development of the APL practitioner.

WHAT IS CAREER?

The literature typically defines career through the concept of *Career Stages*. These are seen as developmental phases of working life, which help to identify the challenges individuals face as they progress from the early stages of their career through to retirement. Career stage theorists often differ in how they identify stages. Some refer to developmental tasks while others refer to chronological age. In addition, some may combine both task and age. The work of a number of stage theorists and their historical contribution to the overall concept of career is now briefly outlined.

Miller and Form (1951) have identified career patterns throughout an individual's lifetime For the adult the most relevant of these is the *Stable work period*. This is characterized by long-term commitment to the kind of work the individual has always wanted or a realization that they may never achieve this. Miller and Form (1951) state that there may be several reasons why an individual may choose to remain in one particular organization or job. These include the advantages of seniority; institutional allegiances; and a strong identification with the values and beliefs of an organization. The emotional tasks the individual faces during the *Stable work period* is concerned with the redefinition of occupational goals that may have been achieved waiting for promotion, or doing work for which the individual is overqualified and which is no longer stimulating.

Dalton *et al.* (1977) have reported the career stages that are relevant to the working adult. For example, as an *Independent specialist* the individual begins to work without supervision to develop his or her abilities and competence. This is achieved by increased specialization. The main task at this stage is to take initiative so that he or she is no longer dependent on their supervisor for decisions about what needs to be done. The next stage is *Mentorship* during this stage the individual becomes concerned not only about his or her own work but also about the work of others. One of the main tasks at this stage is to focus on developing the work of others by coaching. Next is *Sponsorship* the individual becomes involved with the goals and work of larger groups of people. Sponsors ask about the goals of the organization or how the organization fits into the rest of society and may take some initiative in contributing to these. Each stage of Dalton's theory identifies an increasingly broad range and perspective of the work that has to be done, and of the people involved in doing it. However, not all individuals will move through each of the stages identified as some will prefer to remain in the specialist stage, and others may not move from the mentor to the sponsor stage.

Schein (1978) has identified a theory of adult career development. For example, during *basic training and initiation* the individual is socialized into the formal and informal rules and norms of behaviour by others within the organization. This is followed by the *first assignment and promotion* where the individual establishes his or her reputation as possible management material. This is followed by the *second assignment* where the individual continues toward further advancement or begins to plateau. Next is *gaining tenure*, where the individual is admitted to the inner circle of the organization. One of the most important features of Schein's work is the view of the way in which individuals move within organizations. He indicates that individuals have three possible directions of movement. Firstly, *upwards* this is based on the conventional idea of promotion up a hierarchical ladder. Secondly, *inwards* the movement of a person from the *outer circle* at entry to the *inner circle* later on. Thirdly, *around* a person moves from one functional area to another e.g. during job rotation. Each type of promotion may, of course, involve one, two, or all three of these kinds of movement.

Driver (1979) has identified at least three *career types*. Firstly, *Linear* individuals who actively seek to rise in the ranks of an organization. Their drive increases their power and status over time so that they rise quickly and are more successful than those who do not – this is the model of career progression that is seen in most organizations. Secondly, *Steady-state experts* individuals who would rather do the same job over and over again during their careers because their sense of satisfaction comes from doing a job well. This pattern is seen in the professions such as medicine and teaching. Thirdly, *Spirals* individuals who give up power and status for the sake of learning something new. When a Spiral gets close to the top of their profession they get bored and sacrifice status and influence for the sake of doing something different. Each of these career types have something to offer the organization. Linears, bring drive and ambition. Steady-state experts bring competence and skill. Spirals bring fresh ideas and innovation.

Super (1980) indicates that career development takes place across the individual's entire life-span and can be divided into several distinct stages, which include : *Growth* (4–13); *Exploration* (14–24); *Establishment* (25–44); *Maintenance* (45–65); and *Disengagement* (65 and over). However, not everyone progresses through these stages at fixed ages or in the same way. Each stage consists of tasks that will allow individuals to function within that stage before making preparations to move to the next task. Before entering the maintenance stage, Super (1980) suggests that many individuals ask themselves whether they want to remain in the same job and may decide to either 'hang on' or 'let go'. If the individual decides to hang on he or she will enter the maintenance stage. If they decide to let go and change their career they will then reflect on experiences gained in earlier stages to help identify new career prospects and then move forward from there. Those who hold on will maintain what they have, update their skills and knowledge, and attempt to innovate.

Huberrman (1989) has defined the three main stages in a teacher's career. These are the *Novice; Mid-Career;* and *Late Career*. These phases and their intermediate stages are outlined below.

- *The Novice:* during the *Early Novice Stage* the main concern is about survival in a new role. During the *Middle Novice Stage* the main concern is the task of teaching; and during the *Late Novice Stage* the main concern is about the teacher's impact on how students learn.

- *Mid-Career:* teachers in this stage usually feel confident about their professional skills and knowledge and settle into a comfortable and predictable pattern of teaching. Experimental teachers often look for ways to spice up their teaching, trying new approaches and activities in their classrooms. *Taking Stock* teachers reflect on their careers, contemplating their past work and their plans for continued work. Some, may experience a mid-career crisis, look back over their careers and find nothing to look forward to but 'more of the same'.

- *Late-Career: Serenity* teachers with many years of experience are usually comfortable with classroom life and their role in it. *Disengagement:* as they approach retirement, some older teachers start focusing on their lives beyond the classroom, and they begin to distance themselves emotionally from their students.

It is important to note that these phases are not linear, and are often shaped by factors such as personal experiences; the social environment; and organizational influences.

A theory of career for the teaching profession has also been identified by Steffy *et al.* (2001). This theory acknowledges that professional growth happens through a process of reflection and renewal. Steffy identifies the following developmental stages for the teacher. Firstly, the teacher as *novice* this is characterized by the first practicum experience and includes student teaching and internship. Secondly, the teacher as *apprentice* this includes the first two to three years of the new teacher's career. Next, the *anticipatory stage* the new teacher is enthusiastic and eager to perform the tasks of teaching. This eagerness is often confounded by frustrations of the first years of teaching. After the initial years of teaching, the novice or apprentice teacher may move into the next stage of career development, which is the *professional stage* the teacher grows in confidence about his or her teaching ability. Also, respect from students, parents, and other colleagues is evident. Successful completion of this stage leads to the *expert stage* and at this stage the teacher has reached a level of expertise that would meet national certification. Finally, the teacher may enter the *distinguished stage* a teacher who exceeds all expectations of current practice whom is often involved in national educational decision-making (Steffy *et al.*, 2001).

One relatively common feature of both early and contemporary career stage theories is their cyclical pattern. Levinson (1986) for instance, notes that adults experience alternating periods of stability and transition. Also, Miller and Form (1951) argue that many careers are characterized by alternating trial and stable work periods. Similar observations are made by Steffy *et al.* (2001) who describes the frustration of the anticipatory stage and how this evolves into the professional stage of teaching. It is during these periods of stability and instability that individuals examine and then re-examine their values and beliefs with a view to making some kind of career change. Thus, if their careers have been stable for a while, they may begin to get bored and to think about change or introducing some variety. It is from this later perspective, of course, that many individuals become interested in the APL practitioner role i.e. most APL practitioners are experienced teachers or workplace mentors or assessors who already have tenure, but are looking to develop a more specialist role within the organization – either as an APL adviser or an APL assessor.

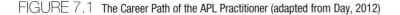

FIGURE 7.1   The Career Path of the APL Practitioner (adapted from Day, 2012)

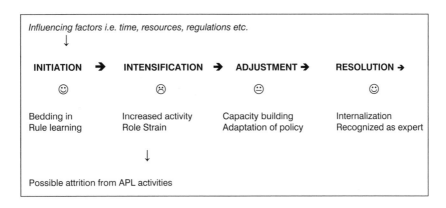

THE CAREER OF THE APL PRACTITIONER

Day (2012) has shown that the practice of prior learning assessment can best be described as a continuous cycle of: *initiation, intensification, adjustment* and *resolution* during which attempts are made by practitioners to resolve the tension that exists between the amount of time and resources available and their choice of assessment method (Figure 7.1).

Each of these stages are now discussed and illustrated.

Stage One: Initiation: during this stage a period of '*bedding in*' occurs, and an appreciation of cultures takes place, during which, the practitioner learns the various rules and regulations of the organization that relate to assessment practice.

Stage Two: Intensification during this stage the workload of the practitioner increases significantly. As a result, the practitioner can experience both *role strain* and *role conflict* as he or she attempts to balance individual APL activity with other organizational commitments. The following example illustrates the feelings of one APL practitioner during this stage: '*I'm allocated time by my job description … this has meant that I continue to teach (in addition to my APL work) … There are no extra APL advisers being (employed) and there has been no change to my working week (hours)*'. The process of *intensification* is critical to the development of the practitioner's career, as it is only when the practitioner successfully makes an adjustment to his or her workload that the risk of attrition from APL activities is minimized.

Stage Three: Adjustment. this stage can best be described as an adaptive activity, undertaken to resolve issues relating to increased demands for assessment while still attempting to maintain some degree of rigor. The following example illustrates the work of one APL practitioner during this stage, who states: '*… we have changed university regulations … we push boundaries within the institute, and change university regulations … to reflect that*'. During this stage roles are redefined and attention is paid to capacity building. Also, regulations, policy and procedures are adapted, and a continuum for assessment practice emerges (Figure 7.2).

Stage Four: Resolution during this stage APL functions become internalized and practitioners may feel liberated as their expertise is recognized by the institution. The following example illustrates the feelings of one practitioner during this stage who states: '*… recognized as experts within the field we've been enabled to take the process forward … I would say that has had a huge impact on our practice.*'

Holistic approach to APL

It is during the *adjustment* phase of the practitioner's career that resources for prior learning assessment become optimized through capacity building and the practitioner adopts an assessment method that is based

FIGURE 7.2 The Stages of Adjustment and Resolution – adapted from Day, 2012

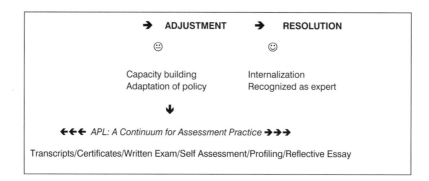

on the individual needs of the learner, rather than the administrative requirements of the organization. Further, the techniques used by the practitioners during this stage of their career tend to be inclusive, rather than exclusive, or specific to, either a *credit based or developmental* approach. Thus, the assessment methods that are used are both diverse and holistic (Day, 2012).

An holistic approach towards APL recognizes the rich diversity of knowledge and learning which a learner can bring to an assessment situation. It promotes diversity and flexibility in the use of assessment methods, according to the individual needs of the learner, and across a continuum for assessment practice and the following comment illustrates the work of one APL practitioner during the adjustment stage of their career. He/she states: '*Self assessment, action planning, reflection, all of these fit very happily within portfolio assessment*' (Day, 2012).

The holistic approach also recognizes the learner's right to actively engage and participate in their assessment through the process of *action planning*. This process is expressed through the following benchmark for practice (Day, 2011).

Activity (II) Agree and review an action plan for demonstration of prior learning:

a) The individual is given accurate advice and appropriate encouragement to enable him or her to form realistic expectations of the value of his or her prior learning.

b) Any outcomes to be achieved are appropriate to the individual's prior learning and future aspirations.

c) Advice to the individual accurately identifies outcomes or agreed-upon criteria which might reasonably be claimed on the basis of prior learning.

d) Opportunities to use evidence from prior learning are accurately analyzed.

e) The individual plan agreed to identifies realistic targets to collect and present evidence of prior learning as efficiently as possible.

f) The individual's motivation and self-confidence is encouraged throughout.

g) If there is disagreement with the advice given, options available to the individual are explained clearly and constructively.

h) The plan is reviewed appropriately with the individual.

The holistic approach is learner focused. The broader purpose of assessment is recognized, which places the learner at the centre of the process (See Chapter 4 for the case study from Canada). This focuses on the preparation of candidates, recognizing what they know, using this information as a basis for future career planning and programme delivery. An holistic approach also recognizes that there are different purposes for the recognition of prior learning and that candidates should be actively involved in deciding the purpose for which they are undertaking prior learning assessment. This purpose may vary, but might include both academic and professional accreditation (See Chapter 3 for the case study from the UK) as well as demonstration of personal competence (See Chapter 6 for the case study from Mauritius). For example, Day (2011) has identified that the key purpose of APL is to:

Review progress and/or assess achievements, so that individuals and organizations can achieve their personal development and/or education and training objectives. This includes assessment of individuals for academic credit and professional certification.

Day (2011)

An holistic approach recognizes that APL should ideally be the first step into a learning programme that will build on the knowledge and skills already recognized. It also locates APL within a broader context of lifelong learning, where individual career planning and flexible programme delivery are part of the services offered. Finally, an holistic approach consciously seeks to address the context and conditions that inform the practice of prior learning assessment these are: educational, economic, political and cultural; and challenges education institutions to re-define curriculum content and qualifications to be more inclusive of the knowledge, skills and values that have been acquired outside the formal education system. For example, Harris (2000:76) suggests that APL may become more inclusive if departments and faculties placed less emphasis on hierarchical forms of knowledge and traditional methods of learning delivery; and placed greater emphasis on problem solving and the application of knowledge to the learner's experience of learning at work.

CONTINUING PROFESSIONAL DEVELOPMENT AND THE CAREER OF THE APL PRACTITIONER

Continuous Professional Development or CPD can be defined as the critical reflection on learning experiences and activities that improve practice, and demonstrate continuous development as a teacher or trainer (Institute for Learning, 2009). These are activities that professionals undertake to keep their knowledge and up-to-date and refreshed. Many professions such as doctors, lawyers and engineers have requirements that members of that profession may have to undertake in regard of CPD, in order to keep their professional status. This may be taken both within work and personal time. However, there can be confusion between the terms: *staff development* and *CPD*. Continuing Professional Development or CPD is that which pertains to the professional activities of the individual, although these may well meet the organizational needs of the institution in which the individual works. Whereas, Staff development activities are normally organized by the employer and while it may meet the needs and wants of the individual, it usually applies to activities that are aimed at meeting the organization's administrative and business needs.

Richter *et al.* (2011:116) indicate how teachers' continuous professional development activities may vary according to career stage. For example, beginning teachers tend to use observations and informal discussions with colleagues to improve their practice, while more experienced teachers are more inclined to use formal meetings for their professional learning. In other words, teachers experience a range of differing learning opportunities across the career cycle.

Richter *et al.* are careful to include both *formal* and *informal* learning opportunities that might deepen and extend teacher's knowledge, beliefs, motivation and self regulatory skills (Richter, 2011:116). They classify formal opportunities as being curriculum based e.g. workshops and courses. Whereas informal opportunities might include more active measures such as teacher conversations; mentoring; study groups, teacher networks and discussion. Further, Richter *et al.* suggest that the attendance of mid career teachers at more formal development programmes is often reduced as the 'pay offs' for this type of activity become smaller as they approach retirement (Richter, 2011;124).

Practitioners of APL are usually experienced workplace supervisors and mentors or assessors, or are faculty members, who are already quite advanced in their career but are looking to develop a more specialist role within their organization, either as an APL adviser or an APL assessor. During the early stages of this career transition it is possible that emergent benchmarks for APL will lend greater clarity and direction to their new role. For example, the following comment highlights the opinion of one practitioner who states that emerging benchmarks for APL will help: '... *organizations identify how practitioners should be prepared for their role and ensures consistency in approach*' (Day, 2012:9).

Also, when practitioners experience *role strain* or *role conflict*. It is possible that emergent benchmarks will lend greater clarity to the role of the APL advisor and assessor by: '... *providing fairly explicit and externally accessible statements that should facilitate quality assurance ...*' (Day, 2012:9). Furthermore, the explicit nature of these benchmarks will enable faculty managers to accurately assess the extent and duration of APL activities, so that appropriate resources can be made available within the institution to support APL activity, thereby minimizing the risk of practitioner attrition. The benchmarks may also be useful in quality assuring the APL process as they will provide a common approach towards assessment, which is both consistent and transparent.

During the *adjustment* phase of the practitioner's career, roles are redistributed and attention is paid to capacity building. During this phase, regulations, policy and procedure are adapted, and a continuum for assessment practice emerges. The following example highlights the usefulness of APL benchmarks during this phase:

> ... *benchmarks serve to advance the self-awareness and reflexivity of practitioners. By encouraging practitioners to probe, reflect on and improve they can help to build up a consensual body of values, criteria and ways of doing things.*
>
> Day (2012:10)

During the *resolution* stage of their career, practitioners feel liberated as their expertise is recognized by peers. The usefulness of benchmarks during this phase is captured by one practitioner who states that they will: '... *enable practitioners to function with a degree of confidence and ensure consistency in all institutions signed up to the benchmark*' (Day, 2012:10). The reader's attention is drawn to the suggestion (here) that there may be a relationship between the use of benchmarks for practice and the ability to practice in a confident manner. In this sense, the agreed benchmarks could become indicators for career success and progression.

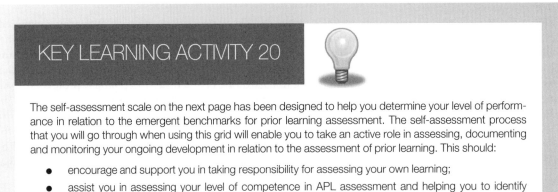

KEY LEARNING ACTIVITY 20

The self-assessment scale on the next page has been designed to help you determine your level of performance in relation to the emergent benchmarks for prior learning assessment. The self-assessment process that you will go through when using this grid will enable you to take an active role in assessing, documenting and monitoring your ongoing development in relation to the assessment of prior learning. This should:

- encourage and support you in taking responsibility for assessing your own learning;
- assist you in assessing your level of competence in APL assessment and helping you to identify gaps in your skills and knowledge;
- assist you in focusing specifically on the APL benchmarks and deciding which of them to pursue by providing evidence of your competence in those areas; and
- promote the design of an individualized learning plan based on your previous experiences and learning related to the benchmarks enabling you to strengthen your existing assessment skills and knowledge, and to fill in any gaps.

The starting point in this process is a candid, thoughtful self-appraisal of your level of competence in relation to the APL benchmarks, and a checklist has been designed to help you identify and compare your skills and knowledge to these. Please check the level of performance which best describes your performance in each of the areas on the self-assessment grid. You can do this by using the following scale.

1   Have no experience with this
2   Have observed this or been oriented to this

3 Can participate in and assist with this

4 Can do this with minimum assistance

5 Can successfully do this without assistance.

Carefully, review each of the functions and activities and their performance indicators. Using the self-assessment scale, record what you think is your present level of performance and understanding. Make notes of possible sources of evidence in the right hand column of any particular tasks, projects, responsibilities, courses, training programmes, self-directed study in which you have participated that may help you to demonstrate competence. You may find that one piece of evidence is strong enough to demonstrate competence in more than one competency area. However, you will probably need more than one piece of evidence to demonstrate adequate performance in any given area. Providing diverse sources of evidence to demonstrate your knowledge and performance is a critical element of the APL process. After completing the self-assessment activity it may be a good idea to pay particular attention to those benchmarks for which you consistently rated yourself as being able to perform with minimum assistance and/or without assistance. Such ratings indicate that these are the areas on which to focus in generating various forms of evidence to support your claim that you possess the required assessment skills and knowledge.

Remember. . . .

Providing appropriate sources and types of documentation (evidence) to support one's level of performance and understanding is a key component of APL Evidence generally falls into two categories; *direct* and *indirect.* Direct evidence refers to products, reports, plans, and performances that you have created and produced. In most cases direct evidence is the strongest evidence to support your claim that you really do have the skills and knowledge that you say you have in relation to the benchmarks. It is important that you collect as much direct evidence related to the benchmarks as possible in support of your claim of competence. Indirect evidence generally refers to information about you and your achievements/competencies. Examples of indirect evidence include letters of validation written on your behalf by employers, supervisors, co-workers, members of professional associations, formal job evaluations, awards, commendations. In many cases, direct evidence or observation of one's skills and knowledge may not be possible due to cost, confidentiality, lack of time, etc. When it is not possible or realistic to provide direct evidence to support one's claim of competence indirect sources of evidence may be used. A flexible combination of direct and indirect evidence is highly desirable and commonly used as an integral part of the APL process. Remember that throughout the assessment process emphasis should be placed on ensuring that diverse sources of evidence are used. This is known as triangulation and the example which follows demonstrates this principle.

Good Luck!

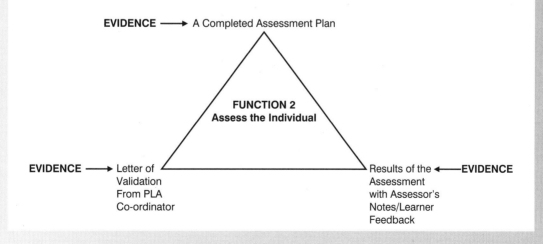

SELF-ASSESSMENT SCALE
BENCHMARKS FOR ASSESSMENT of PRIOR LEARNING (from Day and Zakos, 2000)

FUNCTIONS AND ACTIVITIES

1   Prepare the Individual for Assessment

1. Help the Individual to identify relevant learning.
2. Agree to and review an action plan for demonstration of prior learning.
3. Help the Individual to prepare and present evidence for assessment.

2   Assess the Individual

4. Agree to and review an assessment plan.
5. Judge evidence and provide feedback.
6. Make an assessment decision using differing sources of evidence and provide feedback.

SCALE		1	2	3	4	5	

RATING

1   Have no experience with this
2   Have observed this or been oriented to this
3   Can participate in and assist with this
4   Can do this with minimum assistance
5   Can successfully do this without assistance

FUNCTION 1 – PREPARE THE INDIVIDUAL FOR ASSESSMENT

ACTIVITY	PERFORMANCE INDICATORS	1	2	3	4	5	POSSIBLE EVIDENCE
I. Help the individual to identify relevant learning	a. The individual is given clear and accurate information about the reasons for and methods of, collecting and presenting evidence of prior learning.						
	b. The individual is encouraged to review all relevant and appropriate experience.						
	c. Outcomes or agreed-upon criteria which the individual may currently be able to achieve are accurately identified from a review of their experience.						
	d. The way in which support is given encourages self-confidence and self-esteem in the individual.						
	e. If the individual expresses disagreement with the advice offered, possible alternatives are explained in a clear and constructive manner.						

ACTIVITY	PERFORMANCE INDICATORS	1	2	3	4	5	POSSIBLE EVIDENCE
II. Agree to and review an action plan for demonstration of prior learning	a. The individual is given accurate advice and appropriate encouragement to enable him or her to form realistic expectations of the value of his or her prior learning.						
	b. Any outcomes or agreed-upon criteria to be achieved are appropriate to the individual's prior learning and future aspirations.						
	c. Advice to the individual accurately identifies outcomes or agreed-upon criteria which might reasonably be claimed on the basis of prior learning.						
	d. Opportunities to use evidence from prior learning are accurately analyzed.						
	e. The individual plan agreed to identifies realistic targets to collect and present evidence of prior learning as efficiently as possible.						
	f. The individual's motivation and self-confidence is encouraged throughout.						
	g. If there is disagreement with the advice given, options available to the individual are explained clearly and constructively.						
	h. The plan is reviewed appropriately with the individual.						
III. Help the individual to prepare and present evidence for assessment	a. The individual is provided with suitable support to prepare a portfolio or other appropriate forms of evidence.						
	b. Guidance provided to the individual during evidence preparation encourages the efficient development of clear, structured evidence relevant to the outcomes or agreed-upon criteria being claimed.						

(*continued*)

ACTIVITY	PERFORMANCE INDICATORS	1	2	3	4	5	POSSIBLE EVIDENCE
	c. Liaison with potential assessors establishes mutually convenient arrangements for review of portfolio of evidence, and maintains the individual's confidence.						
	d. Opportunities are identified for the individual to demonstrate outcomes or agreed-upon criteria where evidence from prior learning is not available.						
	e. Any institutional documentation, recording and procedural requirements are met.						
	f. If there is disagreement with the advice given, options available to the individual are explained clearly and constructively.						

FUNCTION 2 – ASSESS THE INDIVIDUAL

ACTIVITY	PERFORMANCE INDICATORS	1	2	3	4	5	POSSIBLE EVIDENCE
I. Agree to and review an assessment plan	a. Any possible opportunities for collecting evidence are identified and evaluated for relevance against the outcomes or agreed-upon criteria to be assessed and their appropriateness to the individual's needs.						
	b. Evidence collection is planned to make effective use of time and resources.						
	c. The opportunities selected provide access to fair and reliable assessment.						

ACTIVITY	PERFORMANCE INDICATORS	1	2	3	4	5	POSSIBLE EVIDENCE
	d. The proposed assessment plan is discussed and agreed with the individual and others who may be affected.						
	e. If there is disagreement with the proposed assessment plan, options open to the individual are explained clearly and constructively.						
	f. The assessment plan specifies outcomes or agreed-upon criteria to be achieved, opportunities for efficient evidence collection, assessment methods and the timing of assessments.						
	g. Requirements to assure the authenticity, currency, reliability and sufficiency of evidence are identified.						
	h. Plans are reviewed and updated at agreed-upon times to reflect the individual's development.						
II. Judge evidence and provide feedback	a. Advice and encouragement to collect evidence efficiently is appropriate to the individual's needs.						
	b. Access to assessment is appropriate to the individual's needs.						
	c. The evidence is valid and can be attributed to the individual.						
	d. Only the agreed-upon criteria and/or outcomes are used to judge the evidence.						
	e. Evidence is judged accurately against all the relevant outcomes or agreed-upon criteria.						
	f. When evidence of prior learning is used, checks are made that the individual can currently achieve the relevant outcome or agreed-upon criteria.						

(continued)

ACTIVITY	PERFORMANCE INDICATORS	1	2	3	4	5	POSSIBLE EVIDENCE
	g. Evidence is judged fairly and reliably.						
	h. Difficulties in authenticating and judging evidence are referred promptly to the appropriate person(s).						
	i. When evidence is not to the agreed standard, the individual is given a clear explanation and appropriate advice.						
	j. Feedback following the decision is clear, constructive, meets the individual's needs and is appropriate to his/her level of confidence.						
III. Make an assessment decision using differing sources of evidence and provide feedback	a. The decision is based on all of the relevant evidence available.						
	b. Any inconsistencies in the evidence are clarified and resolved.						
	c. When the combined evidence is sufficient to cover the outcomes or the agreed-upon criteria, the individual is informed of his/her achievement.						
	d. When evidence is insufficient, the individual is given a clear explanation and appropriate advice.						
	e. Feedback following the decision is clear, constructive, meets the individual's needs and is appropriate to his/her level of confidence.						
	f. The individual is encouraged to seek clarification and advice.						
	g. Evidence and assessment decisions are recorded to meet any PLAR audit requirements.						
	h. Any documentation is legible and accurate, stored securely and referred promptly to the next appropriate stage of the recording/certification process.						

SUMMARY

In this final Chapter the concept of Career and how this applies to the role of the APL practitioner is discussed. The APL Practitioner progresses through a number of significant phases including: *initiation; intensification; adjustment;* and *resolution*. Successful progression through each of these phases is dependent upon the influence of institutional regulations, the time and resources available and the approaches taken towards APL, which (contrary to the literature) may include a credit based *and* developmental approach towards assessment. Practitioners, who are unable to resolve the tensions that exist between institutional regulations, and the time and resources available, withdraw from practice. Practitioners that achieve resolution do so by modifying the rules and regulations of the institution, building capacity for resources and delegation of APL practitioner roles. As a consequence of this adaptive behaviour a more inclusive or holistic approach towards APL emerges.

Further, this chapter has suggested that an holistic approach is supported by a continuum for assessment practice, which identifies a typology of assessment methods associated with a credit or a developmental based approach towards prior learning assessment. For example, credit based approaches include: the use of transcripts, certificates, and products from the work place; while developmental based approaches include: self assessment, profiling, and the use of reflective essays. When using a holistic approach, the APL practitioner will combine a credit based *and* a developmental approach in order to generate evidence for recognition or accreditation.

This Chapter has also indicated that emergent benchmarks for APL will assist the APL Practitioner in transition from novice to expert. In particular, the emergent benchmarks will:

- ensure that assessment of prior learning becomes a defensible process;
- improve accountability and transparency during the assessment process;
- assist education managers to identify what is possible, what is feasible, and what is acceptable for PLA practice;
- ensure consistency of approach towards assessment;
- provide a common understanding and communication between stakeholders; and
- protect the rights of students and assessment service users.

Also, the benchmarks emerging from this study can be used to develop guidelines that might be used by the APL Practitioner during his or her transition from novice to expert. These guidelines include: giving advice and guidance about APL to learners; and assessing and making an assessment of a student's prior learning. Of course, the use of standards setting in education is highly controversial and is anathema to many academics as it has (in the past) been regarded as a form of social control, and has therefore been considered as a potential threat to academic freedom (Day, 2012). More recently, these concerns have been expressed by some academics as an increased demand for performativity (Nixon, 2004). However, there is a *prima facie* case for using the benchmarking process as an adjunct to professional development. This point has been well made by one practitioner who stated: '*Benchmarks serve to advance the self-awareness and reflexivity of practitioners . . .*' (Day, 2012).

Finally, this Chapter has shown how knowledge derived from practice has identified benchmarks for APL that are underpinned by a common set of values and beliefs about the nature and purpose of prior learning assessment. Also, that these emergent benchmarks can be used as a focus for the development of individuals who are involved in undertaking APL activities. This will ensure that the APL process becomes more transparent, open and explicit; and will enable practitioners and their managers to signpost the changing resource requirements for APL capacity building during the critical phase of the APL practitioner's career. This in turn, will ensure that APL practitioners are adequately supported during their transition from novice to expert, and may well assist in minimizing practitioner attrition.

However, there is a more radical view of what professional development might mean for the individual's career, as expressed by Sachs (2003) in her politically motivated account of the: '*Activist Teacher*'. For example, Sachs *describes* how teachers should resist the effects of performativity in order to develop their professional autonomy. Further, Sachs (2003) argues that individuals should take ownership of their profession by creating their own standards, and creating their own milestones for continuing development. With these points in mind, it is suggested that the emergent benchmarks for APL can be used as a mechanism for professionalizing APL activity. Previous attempts to do this have included the development of guidelines and a code of practice for APL e.g. see the work of CAEL, CDLB and SEEC Chapter 1. However, it is important to state that these guidelines and codes of practice appear to be **institutionally focused**, rather than teacher or learner centered. Therefore, it is suggested that the emergent benchmarks ought to be utilized as a pedagogical code of practice for those who perform APL activities. This will provide a framework for assessment practice that is based on a common set of values and beliefs about the nature and purpose of prior learning assessment that have emerged from the reflective (and collective) experience of APL practitioners within the Health and Human Services Professions, both within the UK and Canada. Of course, it is possible that there may be some cultural or philosophical barriers that could impact upon the implementation of the emergent benchmarks as a code of practice. Therefore, it is recommended that disciplines outside the field of Health and Human Services undertake a thorough and systematic review of these, prior to their adoption of the emergent benchmarks. For example, Harris (2000) suggests that it is critical for departments to review their beliefs and assumptions concerning the nature of knowledge and associated mechanisms for teaching, learning and assessment prior to implementing any APL activity. This systematic and analytical approach will ensure that the benchmarks and guidelines discussed in his text can be implemented in a way that is culturally sensitive to the needs of the organization, the learner, and the APL practitioner.

References

About DSST (2012) Get Collect Credi, 2 September. Retrieved from: http://www.getcollegecredit.com/about

Allgoo, K. (2007) *The National Qualifications Framework in Context: The Mauritian Experience*, Paper delivered at the Iveta Conference Mauritius (Unpublished).

Allgoo, K. (2010) *The Introduction of Recognition of Prior Learning in TVET Mauritius – The Mauritian RPL Model, Mauritius Qualifications Authority Report* (Unpublished).

Allgoo, K., Ramdasa, R. and Santokhee, U. G. (2012) 'Recognition and Validation of Prior Learning The Example of Mauritius'. Retrieved August 2012 from: http://www.adeanet.org/triennale/Triennalestudies/subtheme2/2_1_06_ALLGOO_en.pdf

Andersson, P. (2006) 'Different faces and functions of RPL: an assessment perspective', in Andersson, P. and Harris, J. (eds) *Re-theorising the Recognition of Prior Learning*, Leicester: NIACE.

Andersson, P. and Fejes, A. (2005) 'Recognition of prior learning as a technique for fabricating the adult learner: a genealogical analysis on Swedish adult education policy', *Journal of Education Policy* 20: 595–613.

Andersson, P., Fejes, A. and Ahn, S.-E. (2004) 'Recognition of prior vocational learning in Sweden', *Studies in the Education of Adults*, 36: 57–71.

Andersson, P. and Harris, J. (eds) (2006) *Re-theorising the Recognition of Prior Learning*, Leicester: NIACE.

Bamford-Rees, D. (2009) 'Thirty-five years of PLA: we have come a long way', in Hart, D. M. and Hickerson, J. H. (eds) *Prior Learning Portfolios: A Representative Collection*, Dubuque, IA: Kendall/Hunt Publishing.

Betts, D. (2011:10) 'Improving Teaching and Learning through Assessment for Learning', *CPD Matters*. Winter 2011/12. No 2. pp. 9–11

Blower, D. (2000) 'Canada: The Story of Prior Learning Assessment and Recognition' in Evans, N. (Ed.), *Experiential Learning Around the World.: Employability and the Global Economy*, Jessica Kingsley, London. ISBN 1 85302 736 7.

Butterworth, C. (1992) 'More than one bite at the APEL: contrasting models of accrediting prior learning', *Journal of Further and Higher Education* 16(3): 39–51.

Caddye, W. and Hatfield, D. (2011) 'Work-related learning for acute pain management', *Pain News* Summer(37).

CAEL (2010) *Fueling the Race to Postsecondary Success: A 48-institution Study of Prior Learning Assessment and Adult Student Outcomes*, Chicago, IL: CAEL.

CAEL What We Do (2011) CAEL Linking Learning and Work. Retrieved from: http://cael.org/What-We-Do

Canadian Labour Force Development Board (1997) National PLAR Standards, #35, January.

Central Statistics Office (2010) *Digest of Education Statistics 2010*. Retrieved 26 April 2011 from: http://www.gov.mu/portal/goc/cso/report/natacc/edu10/edu2010.pdf

Central Statistics Office (2011) 'National Accounts Estimate (2008–2011) – March 2011 issue Highlights'. Retrieved 26 April 2011 from: http://www.gov.mu/portal/site/cso/menuitem.dee225f644ffe2a338852f8a0208a0c

Challis, M. (1993) *Introducing APEL*, London: Routledge.

CLEP (2012) College Board, 2 September. Retrieved from http://clep.collegeboard.org

Dalton, G., Thompson, P. and Price, R. (1977) 'The four stages of professional careers: a new look at performance by professionals', *Organizational Dynamics*, Summer.

Day, M. (2000a) *Developing Benchmarks for Assessment of Prior Learning and Recognition. Practitioner Perspectives*, Ontario: Canadian Association for Assessment of Prior Learning.

Day, M. (2000b) *Developing Benchmarks for assessment of prior learning and Recognition. Practitioner Perspectives. Canadian Association for assessment of prior learning*, Ontario, Canada. www.capla.ca/bench_en_pl.php

Day, M. (2001a) 'Developing benchmarks for prior learning assessment. Part 1: research', *Nursing Standard* 15(34): 37–44.

Day, M. (2001b) 'Developing benchmarks for prior learning assessment. Part 2: practitioners', *Nursing Standard* 15(35): 38–44.

Day, M. (2002) *Assessment of Prior Learning. A Practitioners Guide*, Cheltenham, Nelson Thornes.

Day, M. (2011) 'Developing benchmarks for prior learning assessment: an exploratory study', *American Journal Health Sciences* 2(2).

Day, M. (2012) 'Developing benchmarks for prior learning assessment. The case for nurse education', *American Journal Health Science* 3(1): 83–96.

Day, M. and Zakos, P. (2000) *Developing benchmarks for prior learning assessment – practitioner perspectives. Guidelines for the Canadian PLAR practitioner*, Ontario: Human Resources Development Canada and the Canadian Association for Prior Learning Assessment.

Department for Business Innovation and Skills (2011) *Higher Education. Students at the Heart of the System*, London: BIS.

Department of Health (1999) *Making a Difference. Strengthening the Nursing, Midwifery and Health Visiting Contribution to Health and Health Care*, London: The Stationery Office.

Department of Health (2004a) *Agenda for Change. Final Agreement*, Leeds: Department of Health Agenda for Change Project Team.

Department of Health (2004b) *The NHS Knowledge and Skills Framework (NHS KSF) and the Development Review Process*, London: Department of Health.

Department of Health (2012) *Liberating the NHS: Developing the Healthcare Workforce*, Leeds: DH

Driver, M. (1979) 'Career concepts and career management in organizations', in Cooper, C. (ed.) *Behavioral Problems in Organizations*, Englewood Cliffs, NJ: Prentice

Fain, P. (2012) 'College credit without college', Inside Higher Ed, 7 May. Retrieved from: http://www.insidehighered.com

Fast Facts (2011) National Center for Education Statistics. Retrieved from: http://nces.ed.gov/fastfacts

Fiddler, M. and Marienau, C. (2009) 'The ten standards for assessing learning', in D. M. Hart and J. H. Hickerson (eds) *Prior Learning Portfolios*, Dubuque, IA: Kendall/Hunt Publishing.

Flint, T. A. (1999) *Best Practices in Adult Learning: A CAEL/APQC Benchmarking Study*, New York, NY: Forbes Custom Publishing.

Flowers, R., and Hawke, G. (2000) The Recognition of Prior Learning in Australia, in Evans, N. (Ed). *Experiential Learning Around the World.: Employability and the Global Economy*. Jessica Kingsley, London. ISBN 1 85302 736 7.

Gamson, Z. F. (1989) *Higher Education and the Real World: The story of CAEL*, Wolfeboro, NH: Longwood Academic.

Harris, J. (2000) *RPL: Power, Pedagogy and Possibility*, Pretoria: Human Sciences Research Council. Pretoria. ISBN 0 7969 1965 8.

Hart, D. M. and Hickerson, J. H. (2009) *Prior Learning Portfolios: A Representative*

Collection, Dubuquense, IA: Kendall Hunt Publishing.

Hemsworth, D. (2007) 'Accrediting prior experiential learning (APEL)', in Brennan, L. and Hemsworth, D. (eds), *Incorporating into Higher Education Programmes the learning people do for and in through work*, Bolton: University Vocational Awards Council.

Higher Education Better Regulation Group (2011) *Professional, Statutory and Regulatory Bodies: An Explanation of their Engagement with Higher Education*, London: HEBRG.

Huberman, M. (1989) 'The professional life cycle of teachers', *Teachers College Record* 91(1): 31–57.

Institute for Learning (2009) *Guidelines for your Continuing Professional Development*, London: Institute for Learning.

Johnson, B. (2002) *Models of APEL and Quality Assurance*, London: Southern England Consortium for Credit Accumulation and Transfer.

Joosten-Ten Brinke, D. *et al.* (2008) 'The quality of procedures to assess credit prior learning: implications for design', *Educational Research Review* 3: 51–65

Kasworm, C. E. and Marienau, A. (1997) *Principles for Assessment of Adult Learning in New Directions for Adult and Continuing Education*, No. 75(Fall). San Francisco, CA: Jose Bass.

Keeton, M. T. (2000) 'Recognizing learning outside of schools in the United States of America,' in Evans, N. (ed.) *Experiential Learning Around the World: Employability and the Global Economy*, London: Jessica Kingsley.

Kenny, G. (2004) 'The origins of current nurse education policy and its implications for nurse educators', *Nurse Education Today* 24: 84–89.

Knowles, M. S. (1980) *The Modern Practice of Adult Education*, Chicago, IL: Association Press.

Knowles, M. S., Holton, E. F. and Swanson, R. A. (2011) *The Adult Learner*. 7th ed., Oxford: Butterworth-Heinemann.

Kolb, D. A. (1984) *Experiential learning experience as a source of learning and development*, New Jersey: Prentice Hall.

Learning Counts (2012) Retrieved from: College credit for what you know: www.learning counts.org

Lenney and Ponton (2007).

Levinson, D. (1986) 'A conception of adult development', *American Psychologist* 41(1): 313.

Lombardi, T., Lovegrove, J., Hatfield, D., Fuggle, S. and Ball, S. (2004) 'NVQs and practice assessment in a pre-registration course', *Nursing Standard* 18(28): 33–37.

Lord, M. (2004) 'Making a difference; the implications for nurse education', *NursingTimes.net* 98(20): 38. Retrieved 16 September 2012 from: http://www.nursingtimes .net/nursing-practice-clinical-research/making-a-difference-the-implications-for-nurse-education/206457.article

Merriam, S. B. and Caffarella, R. (1999) *Learning in Adulthood: A Comprehensive Guide*, 2nd ed., San Francisco, CA: Jossey-Bass.

Merriam, S. B., Caffarella, R. S. and Baumgartner, L. M. (2012) In S. B. Merriam, R. S. Caffarella and L. M. Baumgartner, *Learning in Adulthood: A Comprehensive Guide*, San Francisco, CA: Jossey-Bass.

Merrifield, J. *et al.* (2000) *Mapping APEL: Accreditation of Prior Experiential Learning in English Higher Education*, London: Learning from Experience Trust, Goldsmiths College.

Miller, D. C. and Form, W. H. (1951) *Industrial Sociology*, New York, NY: Harper and Row.

Motaung (2009) 'The nuts and bolts of prior learning assessment in the Faculty of Education of the University of Pretoria, South Africa', *Perspectives in Education* 27(1): 78–84.

Nixon, J. (2004) 'A profession in crisis?', in Hayes, D. (ed.) *Key Debates in Education*, London: Routledge Falmer.

Nursing & Midwifery Council (2004) *Standards of Proficiency for Pre-registration Nursing Education*, London: NMC.

Nursing & Midwifery Council (2008) *Standards to Support Learning and Assessment in Practice*, London: NMC.

Nursing & Midwifery Council (2010a) *Standards for Pre-registration Nursing Education, Section 3: Standards for Education*. Available online at: http://standards.nmc-uk.org/PreRegNursing/statutory/Standards/Pages/Standards.aspx [Accessed 20 December 2012]

Nursing & Midwifery Council (2010b) *Pre-registration Nursing Education in the UK*. Available online at: http://standards.nmc-uk.org/Documents/Pre-registration%20nursing%20education%20in%20UK%20FINAL%2006092010.pdf [Accessed 20 December 2012]

Nursing & Midwifery Council (2010c) *Advice and Supporting Information for Implementing NMC Standards for Pre-registration Nursing Education*, London: NMC.

Nursing & Midwifery Council (2011a) *Using Accreditation of Prior Learning in Existing Pre-registration Nursing, Specialist Community Public Health Nursing Programmes, and in Other Programmes where APL is Permitted*, Circular 01/2011, London: NMC.

Nursing & Midwifery Council (2011b) *The Prep Handbook*, London: NMC.

Ofqual (2009) *GCSEs The Official Student Guide to the System*. Coventry: Office of the Qualifications and Examinations Regulator.

Peruniak, G. and Powell, R. (2007) 'Back eddies of learning in the recognition of prior learning', *Canadian Journal of University Continuing Education* 33(1): 83–106.

Pokorny, H. (2012) 'Assessing prior experiential learning: issues of authority, authorship and identity', *Journal of Workplace Learning* 24(2): 119–132.

Popova-Gonci, V. (2009) 'All work and no PLA makes jack a dull boy', *The Journal of Continuing Higher Education* 57(1): 42–44.

Prozesky, D. (2001) *Community Eye Health*, 2001; 14(38): 27–28.

Quality Assurance Agency for Higher Education (2001) *Benchmark statement. Health care programmes*, Nursing, London: QAA.

Quality Assurance Agency for Higher Education (2004) QAA 2004, *Guidelines for the Accreditation of Prior Learning*, QAA 064 09/04, Gloucester: QAA.

Quality Assurance Agency for Higher Education (2006) *The Code of Practice for the Assurance of Academic Standards in Higher Education, Section 6: Assessment of Students*, September, Mansfield: Linney Direct.

Quality Assurance Agency for Higher Education (2008) *The Framework for Higher Education Qualifications in England, Wales and Northern Ireland*, London: QAA.

Quality Assurance Agency for Higher Education (2011) *UK Quality Code for Higher Education*, Chapter B6: Assessment of students and accreditation of prior learning, Gloucester: QAA.

Quality Assurance Agency for Higher Education (2012) *Recognition Scheme for Subject Benchmark Systems*, 3rd ed., Gloucester: QAA.

Race, P. (2006) *The Lecturer's Toolkit: 3rd Edition* Phil Race, 2006, London, Routledge.

Richter, D., Kunter, M., Klusmann, U., Ludtke, O. and Baumert, L. (2011) 'Professional development across the teaching career: teachers' uptake of formal and informal learning opportunities', *Teaching and Teacher Education* 27: 116–126.

Riffel, M. (2006) *Recognizing the Prior Learning (RPL) of Immigrants to Canada: Moving Towards Consistency and Excellence*, Canadian Association for Prior Learning Assessment.

Retrieved from: http://capla.ca/
Immigrants_to_Canada.php November 2011

Rogers, R. C. (1969) *Freedom to Learn*, Columbus, OH.

Sachs, J. (2003) *The Activisit Teaching Profession*, Buckingham: Open University Press.

SAQA (2012) 'The History of the NQF', The South African Qualifications Authority. Retrieved August 2012 from: http://www.saqa.org.za/show.asp?id=776

Schein, E. (1978) *Career Dynamics*, Reading, MA: Addison-Wesley.

Scott, I. (2010) 'Accreditation of prior learning in pre-registration nursing programmes', *Nurse Education Today* 30, 438–442.

SEEC (1995) *A Quality Code for AP(E)L Issues for Managers and Practitioners. Proceedings of the SEEC National Conference*, 6th December 1995, Southern England Consortium for Credit Accumulation and Transfer, Regents College, London.

Sheckley, B. and Keeton, M. (1995) 'Assessing prior learning: educational benefits', *CAEL Forum and News* 18(1): 9–12.

Simosko, S. (1992) *Get qualifications for what you know and can do: a personal guide to APL*, Kogan Page, London. ISBN 0749404 752

Steffy, B. E. and Wolfe, M. P. (2001) 'A life cycle model for career teachers', *Kappa Delta Pi Record* 38(1): 16–19.

Stern, G. M. (2011) 'Company training programs, what are they really worth?', *CNNMoney*, 27 May. Retrieved from: http://management.fortune.cnn.com/2011/05/27/company-training-programs-what-are-they-really-worth/

Stevens *et al.* (2010)

Super, D. E. (1980) 'A life span, life space approach to career development', *Journal of Vocational Behavior*, 13: 282–298.

Sweygers, A., Soetewey, K., Meeus, W., Struyf, E. and Pieters, B. (2009) 'Portfolios for prior learning assessment: caught between diversity and standardization', *The Journal of Continuing Higher Education* 57(2): 92–103.

Tough, A. (1971) *The Adult's Learning Project: A Fresh Approach to Theory and Practice in Adult Learning*, 2nd ed., Toronto: Ontario Institute for Studies in Education.

Training and Development Lead Body (1995) *National Standards for Training and Development*, Sheffield: Employment Department Group.

Trowler, P. (1996) 'Angels in marble? Accrediting prior experiential learning in higher education', *Studies in Higher Education* 21(1): 17–30.

UKCC (1986) *Project 2000: A New Preparation for Practice*, London: United Kingdom Central Council for Nursing, Midwifery and Health Visiting.

UKCC (1999) *Fitness for Practice: The UKCC Commission for Nursing and Midwifery Education*, London: United Kingdom Central Council for Nursing, Midwifery and Health Visiting.

Vocational Learning Outcomes for Social Worker Programs (2006) Toronto: Ministry of Training, Colleges and Universities.

Wertheim, J. (2009) 'Prior learning assessment today: states of the art', in D. M. Hart (ed.) *Prior Learning Portfolios: A Representative Collection*, Dubuque, IA: Kendal Hunt Publishing.

Whitaker, U. G. (1989) *Assessing Learning: Standards, Principles and Procedures*, Philadelphia, PA Council for Adult and Experiential Learning.

Zakos, P. (2003) *Preparation of a Portfolio for Education, Vocational and Career Planning*, Tyendinga Territory: First Nations Technical Institute.

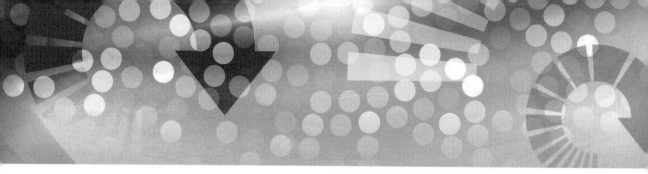

APPENDIX ONE – LEARNING DIARY

INTRODUCTION

A completed learning diary can provide evidence that you have the necessary supporting knowledge and understanding relating to the learning outcomes contained within each Chapter of this book.

When answering each of the: *key learning activities* you should first consider *how* you will learn the new knowledge that is required. For example, you could search out new and relevant information, read it, appraise it and then record it in a meaningful way.

Secondly, you should identify *what* you have learned, taking into account any reading, professional development activities and/or any discussions with others.

You should then state how you will *apply* what you have learned by indicating how any new knowledge will be used to solve a problem or deal with a contingency.

Finally, you should identify the evidence you can use to *demonstrate* that you have the appropriate knowledge. You could do this through discussion with your mentor; by referring to a bibliography or any notes you have written, or any certificates you have achieved.

A sample of a learning diary, together with an explanation of each stage of completion is given on the next page.

SAMPLE LEARNING DIARY

Your Name: _____ **Your Identification No.** _____
Organization: _____ **Name of Mentor:** _____

1. What is my strategy for learning?
After examining the criteria to be achieved within each of the key learning activities in this text you could seek relevant information at the library or have a discussion with a colleague at work, or with a mentor. Keep a record of what you do as this could count as part of the evidence you present in your continuing professional development portfolio.

2. What have I learned?
Based on the information you gained from the above activities, you will need to identify the knowledge you have gained, and indicate how it relates to the criteria to be assessed.

3. How will I apply this knowledge?
State how the knowledge you have gained will be applied to your field of practice. For example, you may use it to solve an existing problem or you could describe how it might be used to solve a potential problem relating to prior learning assessment.

4. What evidence can I demonstrate?
List the possible sources of evidence which demonstrate you have the appropriate knowledge for each of the criteria mentioned in the learning activity. For example; a record of the reading you have undertaken, a copy of any notes you have made, any certificates of attendance you have obtained at training sessions. Don't forget to place a copy of the learning diaries you have completed in your continuing professional development portfolio.

5. Mentor Comments
If you wish you could have your learning confirmed by a third party e.g. your mentor. He/she will need to record whether they agree that you have the necessary supporting knowledge, and understanding and confirm the outcomes you have achieved from undertaking the key learning activities within this text. Your mentor will do this by countersigning your learning diary and making any appropriate comments.

6. Mentors Comments
....
....
....
....
....
....
....
....
....
....
....

Your Signature: _____ Date: _____
Signature of Mentor: _____ Date: _____

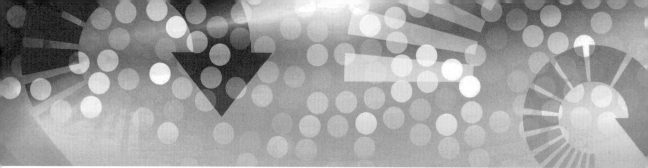

APPENDIX TWO – FEEDBACK ON KEY LEARNING ACTIVITIES

INTRODUCTION

While it is recognized that many of the responses to the key learning activities in each chapter will be individual or context specific, it is important for those who are new to APL to have the benefit of some initial guidance. Please contact the author at: Malcolm.daydayday@talktalk.net to discuss your ideas and responses.

KEY LEARNING ACTIVITY 1, PAGE 8

For example, Trowler (1996) identifies significant tensions underpinning practice, which include: *Cultural*: equality versus elitism – particularly the concept of 'cultural capitalism' as a hidden criterion for access to higher education. *Educational*: education as a product versus education as a process (a similar debate is outlined by Butterworth (1992) in her definition of credit exchange versus developmental models for APL (Chapter 1). *Organizational*: the need to maintain quality to ensure fitness for purpose versus the effects of excessive surveillance on the learning process – in particular alienation rather than internalization of any learning derived through experience. Each of these issues may impact upon the process, or may 'skew' the assessment outcome. These tensions are also present, to some extent, within more traditional forms of assessment.

KEY LEARNING ACTIVITY 2, PAGE 11

You can obtain a copy of the QAA guidelines from: http://www.qaa.ac.uk/Publications/InformationAnd Guidance/Pages/Guidelines-on-the-accreditation-of-prior-learning-September-2004.aspx.

1 and 2. You might want to consider whether the policies you are reviewing are biased towards the institution, if so what impact will this have on the APL process? Also, how transparent are the roles of the learner, the APL Adviser and the APL Assessor?

KEY LEARNING ACTIVITY 3, PAGE 15

1 The QAA (2006:35) indicates that formative assessment has: *'a developmental purpose and is designed to help learners learn more effectively by giving them feedback on their performance and on how it can be improved and/or maintained'*. The QAA (2006:36) states that summative assessment is: *'. . . used to indicate the extent of a learner's success in meeting the assessment criteria used to gauge the intended learning outcomes of a module or programme'*. An APL Practitioner is defined as an individual who utilizes learner-focused activities to diagnose and formatively or summatively assess an individual's prior learning. This includes the work of the APL Adviser and the APL Assessor. If you advise and guide a learner in the development of their portfolio, then someone else should assess the learner's work. This ought to be a subject expert.

2 When establishing their role, APL practitioners should expect to encounter some initial tensions within their organizations. Such tensions may arise in the following situations. *Firstly*, between work colleagues who might question the rationale for selecting one person as an adviser or assessor, rather than another. *Secondly*, between APL assessor and manager, when the assessor negotiates time and space out of normal work activities in order to undertake assessments. *Thirdly*, within individual APL assessors, particularly when they realize that they will be held accountable for their assessment decisions. *Fourthly*, when individuals realize the need to reconcile the demands of being an APL assessor with the demands of being an APL adviser, so that objectivity can be maintained and any potential conflict of interest between the two roles can be avoided or minimized.

KEY LEARNING ACTIVITY 4, PAGE 16

1 See learning activity 3 (above)

2 For example in your plan you could consider whether more than one assessor should be used to carry out the assessment, and whether this should include the need for a subject expert? Do you have regular and direct contact with the learner, if so how might this bias the assessment? Do you work in a different place to the learner, if so how can you be sure about assessing context or contingencies? Is the learner usually supervised, if so could the supervisor be involved in the assessment? Will assessment affect the learner's daily work routine e.g. are there ethical or safety issues to consider Would your assessment methods place an unfair burden on the learner? Could any of your assessment documentation be integrated with other organizational systems such as performance appraisal, training and development plans, or total quality management procedures?

KEY LEARNING ACTIVITY 5, PAGE 17

1, 2 and 3. There are no right or wrong answers to these questions. However, if you review your answers to the previous learning activities in this Chapter this will help you to decide whether your organization wishes to develop a generic APL role, which includes giving advice and assessing. Or, whether a specialist assessor role is more appropriate where the learner is advised by an APL adviser but assessed by a subject expert. If a generic role is deemed to be appropriate you should consider how bias can be minimized during the assessment process e.g. some organizations who use generic practitioners have faculty examination boards who assess the learners portfolio before credit is awarded. These boards are comprised of individuals who are subject experts who have not previously worked with the learner.

KEY LEARNING ACTIVITY 6, PAGE 26

Kenny's (2004) paper explores the prevailing powers in society at the time of the *Fitness for Practice* report (UKCC, 1999). Nurse education was subject to scrutiny because the UK Government and the National Health Service (NHS) were concerned that newly qualified nurses were not fit for purpose. There was also a need to control public spending and so economic forces drove the direction of higher education (HE). Knowledge could be acquired through key skills and this favoured the argument for competency-based approaches to learning. NHS service providers effectively dictated the flow of students so that there would be an adequate labour force. Kenny (2004) talks of this being described as a 'society-centred model of preparation'. Nurse educators were seen as out of touch and so partnerships between HE and employers were never going to be equal. Nurse educators wanting to maintain nursing values and promote holistic care were marginalized in an era that saw skills competency as more important. The entry gate was also widened to increase numbers of nursing students and maintain workforce demands.

There are a number of parallels with the present day; the NHS is undergoing major reform in austere times and has to make unprecedented savings. Nurses who qualified with (and without) a diploma qualification are becoming graduates in order to compete with the new style nurse prepared to degree level at the point of registration. This process can be protracted and costly especially if individuals struggle with the academic level. Less funding is available to finance staff to 'top up' to degree level and so APL can be an attractive option to save both time and money. It also encourages a developmental approach to learning with opportunity to reflect on technical competence. Meanwhile the argument for a more compassionate and caring workforce gathers momentum and nursing values have gained increasing importance within curricula.

KEY LEARNING ACTIVITY 7, PAGE 27

The answer to this activity will depend on what you selected from the menu. Some colleges have more details than others, for example, searching on the Sussex Downs College (Lewes Campus) web pages under Access to Higher Education you find:

- You have to be over 19 years of age.
- The course is approximately 34 weeks in duration.
- It runs during the daytime or in the evening.
- Core elements include Communication and Learning Skills, Maths, Critical Thinking, Academic Literature, using Information Technology for Academic Work.
- Health topics include Health and Society, Health Studies, Introduction to Psychology, Life Systems, Homeostasis, Anti-discriminatory Practice and Science equivalence (if necessary).

The course is QAA approved and validated by the Open College Network.

KEY LEARNING ACTIVITY 8, PAGE 29

This activity enables you to explore two websites with regard to career structure and maintaining professional registration. The first is Flying Start NHS England. The suggestion to find the *Career Pathways* menu should take you to resources to meet the following learning outcomes:

- Explore the possible short and longer term options for your career development.
- Understand the role of NHS KSF in assisting your career pathway.
- Develop the skills to effectively manage your career.
- Identify the available resources to assist your career pathway.

The PREP handbook on the NMC website highlights that you must have worked in some capacity of your registered qualification for a minimum of 450 hours over the previous three years. Also, undertaken at least 35 hours of learning activity relevant to your practice during the three years prior to renewal of your registration.

KEY LEARNING ACTIVITY 9, PAGE 31

This activity refers to the NMC 2004 *Standards of proficiency for pre-registration nursing education*. Some of the answers to the activity questions are contained within the text of the chapter.

Where previous academic or experiential learning is recognized the minimum length of the course is two years (3066 hours). If that prior experience includes an existing registration with the NMC, there is no required minimum length, (standard 4).

Guidance on appropriate prior learning and experience includes National Vocational Qualifications at level 3, Cadet Nurse Schemes, Health Care Assistant programmes where learning has been assessed and relevant degrees. The definition of advanced standing is:

Advanced standing is where a student enters a programme, normally beyond the initial start point, as a result of the award of AP(E)L or prior registration, thus being able to undertake a shortened programme

NMC (2004:11)

Note that in 2004 the NMC differentiated between prior learning and experiential learning by including the 'e' in brackets within the acronym AP(E)L.

For quality assurance purposes, all evidence should be available to show how common foundation programme outcomes and proficiencies within the branch standards are met.

KEY LEARNING ACTIVITY 10, PAGE 32

This activity refers to the NMC 2010 *Standards for Pre-registration Nursing Education*. The answers to the questions are contained within the text of the chapter with a more in depth consideration of the requirements.

KEY LEARNING ACTIVITY 11, PAGE 40

The primary differences between a holistic approach and a technical approach in PLAR are:

1 A holistic approach emphasizes both a process and a product. The process involves working with an advisor to reflect on one's prior life and work experiences and the product is the creation of a portfolio to demonstrate one's learning. The technical approach is less concerned about process and more focussed on product (e.g., academic transcripts, trade certificates, post secondary diplomas).

2 The relationship between the advisor and the PLAR candidate is critical in the holistic approach as it involves trust, honesty, perseverance, encouragement and confidentiality. The advisor must possess strong interpersonal skills and a sound knowledge of interviewing techniques, PLAR procedures and institutional policies. The relationship element in the technical approach is minimal, inconsequential or, in some instances, non-existent. Generally it involves providing basic information outlining what steps the candidate must follow to prove competence and what documentation they must provide as evidence.

KEY LEARNING ACTIVITY 12, PAGE 43

When interviewing a PLAR candidate it is useful to use both **closed questions** to acquire specific, factual information (e.g., name, address, workplace, schools attended, etc.) and **open-ended questions** that elicit more than a short answer or a Yes/No response. An example of an open-ended question is 'Can you tell me more about that experience?'

Here are a few sample questions used in initial PLAR interviews:

1 So what brings you here today?

2 How can we help you?

3 Can you tell me about some of your past work experience?

4 Where do you hope the PLAR process will lead you?

KEY LEARNING ACTIVITY 13, PAGE 44

After the initial interview, getting started is sometimes the most difficult part. The advisor can ask the candidate where they would like to begin by either reflecting back on their past experiences or looking ahead to where they want to go. If reflecting back is their preference, then working on the Chronological Record or the Life History paper are useful exercises to engage in. If looking ahead is a preferred starting point, then creating a Goals Paper, comprised of short term and long term Education/Career and Personal goals, is important.

Regardless of which process the candidate chooses, provide an outline of the exercise, describe the steps to completing it, show them an example of one, and offer to review a draft of their work once they've finished it.

KEY LEARNING ACTIVITY 14, PAGE 45

There are two broad types of documentation or evidence in PLAR: direct and indirect evidence. Direct evidence includes documents produced/performed by the candidate such as plans, reports, proposals, research data/findings, books written, photographs, videos, demonstrations, models, etc. Indirect evidence includes documents provided by third parties such as reference letters, awards, certificates, diplomas, newspaper and magazine articles, etc.

In PLAR, proving one's knowledge, skill and competence is the primary purpose of the work. The concept of triangulation involves presenting three diverse pieces of documentation to prove competence in a particular subject area. This could include both direct and indirect evidence.

KEY LEARNING ACTIVITY 15, PAGE 47

Assisting candidates to overcome barriers or challenges is a key function of the PLAR Advisor. Here are a few tips to assist in reducing barriers:

1 Check in frequently with the candidate about how the process is going.

2 Offer more support and encouragement in the beginning as the need is usually greater then than towards the end of the PLAR process.

3 If the candidate gets stuck or appears to be discouraged, try to determine what the cause is and explore options together to get unstuck or to simply move on to another exercise (and possibly return to the difficult one at a later time).

4 Identify and share with the candidate their strengths.

5 Respond to the candidate's questions and concerns immediately. Ongoing feedback is essential.

KEY LEARNING ACTIVITY 16, PAGE 61

For the learner

There is no one correct answer for the development of an educational plan. It is not unusual for adult learners to have several options for degree completion and thus, may need to explore designing several educational plans before they select the plan best for them. For example, a learner may need to decide to complete a degree in hospital administration or business management. Examining each degree program and the planning questions will assist the learner with gathering information to make an informed choice. They can use that information to select the degree program that fits with their career goals and be completed in the timeliest manner. The process begins with the following checklist.

- List career and educational goals.
- Explore degree options related to career goals.
- Examine courses needed to complete the degree.
- If a learner has previous college credits at the college/university or transfer credit from another institution, how does this learning apply to the degree?
- Examine learning from prior experiences and explore what courses learner might be able to receive credit.
- Are there multiple prior learning methods available to challenge the courses that need to be completed by the learner? What are they?
- Discuss with the learner which methods would be more efficient given their learning styles, preferences and availability of documentation to support their requests.
- List the courses that will be challenged using the prior learning method.
- What courses are needed to complete the degree program? Are there instructional options available to complete the course, i.e in-class, distance learning, independent study, etc.
- Select the best method to complete each new courses and prepare a time line for completion.

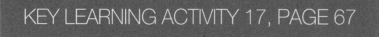

KEY LEARNING ACTIVITY 17, PAGE 67

1 After having reviewed the Background of this Chapter identify the opportunities and benefits of implementing RPL in the Mauritian Education and Training System?

2 Do you believe that the RPL system is based on the 'one size fits all' approach?

- *By adopting RPL within the Mauritian Education and Training system, access has been rendered more flexible. People, who were previously left out of the system due to the lack of academic or formal education, now have the possibility to validate their experiences – be it informal or non-formal – into nationally recognized certificates. With clear learning pathways, more people can re-embark on training programmes and participate in lifelong learning. Being personally and socially empowered, the Mauritian labour force will be well-equipped to face future challenges and more importantly help sustain the island's economy.*

- *The RPL model cannot be based on the 'one size fits all' strategy. The model has to be developed and designed keeping in mind the country's socio-economic context. Although common benchmarks can be adopted, each country will have to put in place a structure corresponding to the demands of the country and its people.*

KEY LEARNING ACTIVITY 18, PAGE 72

1 According to you what are the qualities of Facilitators and their role within the RPL process?

Facilitators have a key role to play within the RPL process. Their duty is essentially to offer support to the Learner and to act as a guide to the latter. In short, the Facilitator supports the learner in the reflection of their prior experiences in order to identify potential evidences of learning which can be matched against the competences of National Qualifications. However, while being in direct contact with the Learner, Facilitators must strictly refrain from personally involving themselves in the actual development of the portfolio. Their qualities must be such that they can effectively communicate with the Learner and have the knowledge and skills required in ensuring that the learner knows how to generate the evidence of learning without self-involving themselves in the gathering of evidences. The Facilitator must be an expert in the field of the RPL demand, as he/she will have to provide information about the qualification, competences and experiences required. This is a crucial point as the Facilitator has as task to not only guide the learner but to help keep their expectations realistic while keeping them grounded in the gathering of evidences.

KEY LEARNING ACTIVITY 19, PAGE 73

Discuss the role of Stakeholders in the implementation of RPL?

Given the nature of RPL, stakeholders help define and stimulate the growth of RPL within a set education and training system. By involving stakeholders within the implementation process, issues such as credibility and legitimacy are automatically improved. In effect, the collaboration of stakeholders is vital to the sustenance of RPL. Consolidating links with both internal and external stakeholders will strengthen the rationale behind RPL, enabling more people to partake in the system and to adopt it. Such steps are critical to building confidence in recognition processes and to meeting learner needs. In short, consolidating a national approach to RPL.

Glossary

Assessment   the Quality Assurance Agency for Higher Education (QAA) indicates that: '... *assessment describes any processes that appraises an individual's knowledge, understanding, abilities or skills*' (QAA 2006:4).

Assessment of Prior Learning or APL   is a systematic process that involves the identification, documentation, assessment and recognition of learning (i.e. skills, knowledge and values). This learning may be acquired through formal and informal study including work and life experience, training, independent study, volunteer work, travel, hobbies and family experiences.

APL Practitioner   an individual who utilizes learner or client-focused assessment activities to formatively or summatively assess an individual's prior learning, either for academic credit or recognition of competence. This includes the work of the Advisor. It also includes the work of the Assessor – who is often but not exclusively, a subject matter expert from faculty. It may also include the work of the Co-ordinator – if he or she is directly involved in the guidance and assessment of individuals.

Authentic   evidence that can be directly attributed to a learner is said to be authentic.

Benchmark   a reference or marker of best practice.

CAEL   Council for Adult and Experiential Learning. A USA based organization which has been highly influential in establishing guidelines and protocols for international APL practice. Contact: www.cael.org/

CAPLA   Canadian Association of Prior Learning Assessment. A national network of APL practitioners for Canada. Contact: http://capla.ca/

Client focused assessment   any assessment activity which primarily focuses on the individual needs of a learner e.g. his or her culture, personal learning style or language preference.

Current   evidence which is up-to-date is said to be current.

Formative assessment   developmental and ongoing, i.e. its purpose is to identify for and with learner's areas in need of improvement.

Institutionally focused assessment   any assessment activity which primarily focuses on the needs of an institution or organization, e.g. the development of articulation agreements between and across institutions and departments etc.

Learning Diary   a reflective document maintained by the learner in order to demonstrate underpinning knowledge, as well application to practice (see Appendix One).

NVQ   National Vocational Qualifications. A nationally recognized UK credential now replaced by QCF awards, certificates and diplomas.

QCF   the UK Curriculum and Qualifications Framework, which encompasses both Further and Higher Education.

Reliability   the degree to which an assessor's opinion may match that of another assessor in the same situation, with the same learner, using the same criteria. Reliability can be improved if advisors and assessors are able to meet on a regular basis to discuss and agree assessment requirements in order to achieve some standardization and consistency of approach. This is an activity which is often overseen by the APL Co-ordinator.

SEEC   is a highly respected authority in the existing and developing field of Credit Accumulation and Transfer (CATS) at higher education levels. Contact: http://www.seec.org.uk/

Simulation   an assessment method which is based on direct observation of any performance other than the learner's normal, naturally-occurring work activity. Simulation can be used as an assessment method if safety or confidentiality are an issue in the workplace. They may also be used if work cements for students are limited e.g. use of demonstration workshops or clinical laboratories.

Sufficiency if all of the criteria within each of the specified outcomes or competencies have been met then the evidence is said to be sufficient e.g. the need to demonstrate both range and diversity of practice, or to demonstrate contingencies.

Summative assessment undertaken to judge a learner's knowledge, skills and values at a defined point in time for the purpose of awarding a final grade, or granting some credit.

Triangulation the use of several (and different) assessment methods to cross validate (or confirm) the performance and underpinning knowledge of a learner against the required competency or outcome.

Validity an assessment should only be based upon the required outcomes or competencies and their associated criteria. An assessment is said to be valid if the assessor refers only to these stated criteria. Validity can be improved if the assessment criteria are explicit and made clear to the Adviser, Assessor and the learner.

Validation Letter a letter from a knowledgeable and competent third party, which can be used to support an individuals claim to competence.

Index